Medical Decision Making
A Physician's Guide

Medical Decision Making

A Physician's Guide

Alan Schwartz, Ph.D.

Departments of Medical Education and Pediatrics
University of Illinois at Chicago

George Bergus, M.D.

Department of Family Medicine
University of Iowa

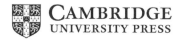
CAMBRIDGE
UNIVERSITY PRESS

CAMBRIDGE UNIVERSITY PRESS

Cambridge, New York, Melbourne, Madrid, Cape Town, Singapore, São Paulo, Delhi

Cambridge University Press
The Edinburgh Building, Cambridge CB2 8RU, UK

Published in the United States of America by Cambridge University Press, New York

www.cambridge.org
Information on this title: www.cambridge.org/9780521697699

First published 2008

Printed in the United Kingdom at the University Press, Cambridge

A catalog record for this publication is available from the British Library

Library of Congress Cataloging-in-Publication data
Medical decision making : a physician's guide / Alan Schwartz, George Bergus.
    p. ; cm.
  Includes bibliographical references and index.
  ISBN 978-0-521-69769-9 (pbk.)
    1. Medicine—Decision making. I. Schwartz, Alan, 1970- II. Bergus, George.   II.Title.
  [DNLM: 1. Decision Making.   2. Physician—Patient Relations.   3. Ethics, Medical.
4. Informed Consent.   5. Patient Participation.   6. Treatment Outcome.
W 62 M4891 2008]

R723.5.M39   2008
610—dc22   2008010488

ISBN   978-0-521-69769-9 paperback

Contents

Part V Beyond the individual

Foreword

This lucid, well-written book fills a distinct gap in the literature on decision making in the health professions, especially medicine and nursing. What is this gap? And how does this book address it?

Introductory presentations of medical decision making typically begin with how to assess the accuracy of clinical evidence, especially diagnostic tests, and move on to drawing inferences. Making diagnostic judgments is conceptualized as a problem of updating opinion with imperfect information, and Bayes's theorem is the method to solve the problem. Probability and uncertainty are highlighted and Bayes's theorem is presented in one form or another. Other books are intended as graduate texts for health professionals who wish to practice decision analysis or do research using statistical decision theory. This book is positioned somewhere between those two poles.

Instead of starting with diagnostic testing, it begins with the problem of determining goals and objectives of medical care and with methods for assessing values and the quality of life. It does not neglect probability, uncertainty and how they can be effectively discussed with patients, but it puts values, utility assessment and choice on center stage. Interestingly, it does not get to Bayes' theorem and diagnostic testing until better than halfway through the text. By that time, the reader should have a very good idea of how concepts and principles of medical decision making extend well beyond the setting of diagnosis with which the field arguably began. Importantly, it shows that a scientific approach to medical decision making is not limited to technical rationality, but can pay close attention to the values and goals of thoughtful clinical practice.

Within these pages, all of the major topics in medical decision making are covered at a level of detail appropriate for a text intended for physicians and other health professionals who do not intend to specialize in the area but who want to know, in broad terms, what it is about. The topics include: 1) the role of values in many decisions and how they can be quantified for systematic decision making; 2) decision making with multiple, sometimes competing objectives, and thinking about trade-offs; 3) decision analysis, including sensitivity analysis, and ways of visualizing decisions, including decision trees and influence diagrams; 4) cost-effectiveness analysis, including measuring the quality of health outcomes (quality-adjusted life years); and 5) psychology of judgment and decision making. Findings of three decades of research in decision psychology are especially well integrated into the exposition. It concludes with chapters on family involvements in clinical decisions and other ethical issues.

Recently, medical decision making has been treated largely as an adjunct to evidence-based medicine. This book emphasizes a very different perspective that is, in my opinion, much needed: evidence-based medicine is discussed in a few pages, while value and quality-of-life issues are much more prominent.

The book makes a sustained effort to address the needs and concerns of learners and novices in the field. It is not a graduate text in any of the topics discussed. Mathematical formalisms and notation are kept to a minimum to increase its appeal to health-care professionals. The reasons why we should care about a particular question introduce the exposition of the methods used to approach it. The connections between clinically realistic situations and fundamental concepts and theories are repeatedly emphasized. So if one is looking for a book effectively written at a level appropriate for physicians and other health professionals who want an overview of the territory, it is in your hands. It deserves a wide audience.

Arthur S. Elstein, Ph.D.
October, 2007

Preface

Decision making is a key activity – perhaps the key activity – in the practice of health care. Although physicians acquire a great deal of knowledge and many specialized skills during their training and through their subsequent practice, it is in the exercise of clinical judgment and its application to specific decisions facing individual patients that the outstanding physician is distinguished. This has become even more true as patients have been increasingly welcomed as partners in increasingly complex medical decisions, in what has been termed "shared decision making."

Medical decision science is a field that encompasses several related pursuits. As a normative endeavor, it proposes standards for ideal decision making. As a descriptive endeavor, it seeks to explain how physicians and patients routinely make decisions, and has identified both barriers to, and facilitators of, effective decision making. As a prescriptive endeavor, it seeks to develop tools that can guide physicians, their patients, and health care policymakers to make good decisions in practice.

Although there have been decades of research and theory on the judgment and decision making of physicians and patients, this "basic science" of the decision process has too often been unknown outside the province of the academic medical center. Just as a substantial crevasse separates the theoretical geneticist from the general practitioner who could benefit from new developments in genetics and genomics, a similar canyon gapes between the decision scientist and the community physician.

The goal of this book is to bridge that gap – to provide a practical, conceptual, clinical translation of the work of decision theorists, analysts, and psychologists – and to do so in a way that will be interesting and useful to a busy physician.

We come to this book with several fundamental beliefs. Our first fundamental belief is that a large majority of clinical decisions are variations of basic patterns of decision problems that are similar across specialties, and amenable to the same basic classes of conceptual tools. All carpenters apply a common set of tools to a common raw material. A master carpenter, however, produces valuable and unique pieces by critically evaluating the distinctive grain of a piece of wood, carefully choosing which tools are appropriate, and skillfully applying those tools to best effect. A master clinician similarly achieves great results for patients by considering each patient as a unique individual and selectively applying conceptual tools in a skillful manner.

Our second fundamental belief is that making good decisions is more important in practice than making perfect decisions. As a result, the treatment of decision science in this book is both at a high conceptual level and necessarily abridges some of the finer grained mathematical distinctions that are of great interest to decision scientists. For readers who wish to explore the ideas we present in greater detail or mathematical rigor, we provide references to key works in modern decision theory.

Our third fundamental belief is that many clinical decisions require input from both physicians and patients, but physicians and patients are not interchangeable. Each brings a unique perspective and unique information that is largely inaccessible to the other – a point that is often made when physicians write about their own experiences as patients. A theme of this book is to consider how much and what kind of information must be provided by the patient in different types of decisions to make the decision process successful.

Our fourth fundamental belief is that the practice of medicine and health care policy are inseparably linked. Acts of clinical care are influenced by public policy and social context; in many important cases, acts of clinical care may even be expressions of policy. When health care demand exceeds resources, when access to care is difficult or inequitable, or when other factors conspire to constrain physicians' abilities to provide excellent care, they often become advocates not only for their individual patients, but for the health of their society. As these circumstances are common in both the developed and developing world, this book also introduces ideas in decision science that go beyond choices that affect an individual patient to those that impact the patient's family, community, and society.

This is a book for physicians and other smart, busy, independent-minded people with a deep concern for the health and well-being of others. We are medical educators, and as such, we know that the lecture is the least effective way of conveying information. Accordingly, this book is organized around typical clinical cases in a variety of specialties and is designed to encourage the reader to reflect on the application of the concepts presented to their own clinical practice. Where possible, chapters are self-contained, allowing the reader to approach the book in the order most useful for them and to use it as a convenient reference; where chapters must refer to earlier chapters, this is clearly noted. A brief synopsis of each chapter follows.

Part I

Goals of medical care

Chapter 1 – Goals and objectives

Your patient has just been diagnosed with lung cancer, and you know that she will face many decisions about her treatment and will look to you for information and guidance. Good decisions are characterized first and foremost by good decision processes – approaches designed to increase the likelihood and degree to which important goals are achieved. Before any choices can be considered, decision makers should clarify their goals and objectives. This chapter presents a typology of goals and how they operate in medical decisions, together with suggestions for how you can facilitate your patient's clarification and refinement of their goals.

Part II

Valuing health

Chapter 2 – Components of health

Your patient has diabetes and is facing decisions about how intensively to manage his disease. He needs to better understand the health states that may face him in the future, each of which is multifaceted. Most health outcomes involve several different dimensions of health. Moreover, not all dimensions are equally important. Here we encounter a basic paradox of medical judgment: while only patients can truly know how much importance to give to each dimension of health, their experience is nearly always more limited than that of their physician, who may have treated scores or hundreds of patients with similar conditions and seen the results of their decisions. This chapter discusses health dimensions and subdimensions that are commonly used to measure quality of life and introduces processes for patients and physicians to identify the importance of health dimensions and evaluate the likely range of outcomes on each dimension.

Chapter 3 – The overall health state

Your diabetic patient has considered how his future health states might impact him across several dimensions but is reluctant to limit himself to those dimensions. Concerned about the possibility of failing to consider important facets of health or how different facets of health might interact, he wants to know how he might evaluate his overall health state. This chapter demonstrates and compares two methods for the identification and evaluation of health states as whole, the decompositional and holistic approaches.

Chapter 4 – Quality and quantity

Your patient has degenerative osteoarthritis in her knee and is considering total knee replacement surgery. Her decision is typical of a large group of decisions that feature trade-offs between future quality and quantity of life, particularly over the natural history of a degenerative disease. How should she think about her future quality of life and consider the course of her health over her lifetime?

Part III

Understanding uncertainty

Chapter 5 – Embracing uncertainty

A public health screening leads a patient to consult you about his cholesterol levels and ask whether he's likely to have a heart attack and whether a dietary supplement might reduce his risk. Uncertainty makes both patients and physicians nervous, but is a fundamental feature of medicine. This chapter shows how understanding different types of uncertainty can help put patients at ease and guide physicians to identify the most important questions to consider in planning a workup or treatment program.

Chapter 6 – Chance and choice

Your patient has been diagnosed with prostate cancer and is considering which of the several courses of treatment he should follow, if any. Each offers some hope of keeping the cancer in remission, but each also presents risks of serious side effects. Most medical decisions present the possibility of several possible outcomes, with no certainty about which will actually occur. This chapter introduces tools for evaluating and comparing such options by combining information about the probabilities of outcomes with insights about the values of outcomes.

Chapter 7 – Confidence

A physician describes his hypertensive patient's 10-year risk of heart attack, and the patient asks how confident the physician is in his estimate of the risk and in the likely benefit of treatment. Determining the best choice to achieve a goal is not always enough to complete a decision. Often, a physician, policy maker, or patient is also concerned with how confident they should be that the recommended choice is superior to other options, and the conditions under which another option would be recommended instead. This chapter discusses both subjective and statistical confidence.

Part IV

Developing information

Chapter 8 – Visualizing decisions

A couple are unsure about what kind of prenatal Down's syndrome screening strategy they should choose, and ask for your assistance in understanding the decision. One of the most powerful classes of decision aids are tools for making options, outcomes, and attributes visually comprehensible. This chapter introduces several different kinds of decision visualization and communication tools and develops a vocabulary and taxonomy for creating and evaluating new tools. Particular attention will be paid to tools for constructing choice sets, weighing and evaluating attributes, and representing the structure of decisions.

Chapter 9 – The power of information

Another couple facing the prenatal Down's syndrome screening decision has chosen to undergo amniocentesis, but has additional questions about the risks of the procedure and their own preferences for outcomes. One of the available options in many decisions is to gather more information. We can conceptualize the usefulness of additional information by considering how much a decision recommendation could be improved if that additional information were available. However, additional information often comes at a cost. This chapter provides both a conceptual and simplified mathematical introduction to the use of information in decisions and offers the clinician strategies for determining which information should be obtained in a decision and when. The chapter also discusses evidence-based medicine and the development of clinical trials.

Chapter 10 – Screening and testing

In many clinical decisions, the most ready source of additional information is diagnostic testing. Diagnostic tests include not only laboratory tests, but also other sources of information about diagnosis, such as history and physical examination. Many physicians, however, do not understand how diagnostic tests are developed or how to determine the value of the information they provide. The chapter case illustrates these concepts by considering the diagnosis of *Helicobacter pylori* infection in an adolescent girl with iron-deficiency anemia. Diagnostic testing strategies involving multiple tests in series or parallel are explained. This chapter also discusses psychological heuristics associated with diagnosis and conditions under which such judgments are helpful or misleading.

Part V

Beyond the individual

Chapter 11 – Family matters

Physicians are accustomed to making recommendations for others; patients, however, face additional and often unfamiliar complexities when they find themselves in a position of "agency" – responsible for decisions that affect the health of a child, an aged parent, or an incapacitated spouse. How can physicians guide patients in these situations? This chapter reviews research on how medical decision making for another differs from decision making for the self and develops recommendations for physicians whose patients seek guidance on agency. Two chapter cases illustrate applications of these recommendations: in one, a married couple consults you about prostate cancer treatment for the husband; in the other, a woman asks about assuming decision-making responsibility for her mother, who has mid-stage Alzheimer's disease.

Chapter 12 – Public health

In the United States, physicians have traditionally focused their attention on the clinical treatment of their patients with little concern for matters of public health or the cost of medical care, but this focus has changed dramatically in the last 20 years. In other countries, physicians have always been responsible for the broader health of their societies. This chapter introduces elements of decisions involving public health. First, it considers the problem of the aggregation of value: how should society place a value on health states that may be evaluated differently by different patients? Research in the area of utility aggregation and contingent valuation is reviewed. Second, the chapter discusses direct and indirect costs and savings associated with medical care and briefly explains guidelines for the measurement of medical costs to society. Finally, the chapter combines the two by introducing cost-effectiveness analysis as a model for allocating a budget to public health programs and reviews the cost-effectiveness of several kinds of public health and medical interventions in current use. The chapter case illustrates the concepts by presenting research on the cost-effectiveness of routine hepatitis A vaccination of young children.

Chapter 13 – Social values

The final chapter once again takes up decision goals and objectives, but from the perspective of shared social values and ethical norms. This chapter makes explicit a variety of often implicitly accepted priority rules for decisions that involve rationing care (triage, the "rule of rescue", cost-effectiveness) and uses organ donation and transplant as a case illustration. It also considers the application of values and goals beyond simply improving a patient's health, such as the value of research that is not expected to be beneficial (e.g., Phase I drug trials).

Appendix

The appendix summarizes the questions for clinical practice that arise from each of the chapters. It may be used as a tool for reflection or a quick guide to questions that might be considered in helping patients make decisions about their health.

We welcome feedback from our readers and the opportunity to continue the conversation of this book on our web forum at www.makingmedicaldecisions.com.

Acknowledgments

We would like to thank the many colleagues whose work has been inspirational for us and from whose guidance we have benefited, including George Lakoff, Barbara Mellers, Danny Kahneman, Alan Cooke, Arthur Elstein, David Meltzer, Gordy Hazen, Suzanne Poirier, Georges Bordage, Les Sandlow, Jerry Niederman, Jordan Hupert, Robert Hamm, and the faculty of the Departments of Medical Education and Pediatrics at the University of Illinois at Chicago and Department of Family Medicine at the University of Iowa. This book was prepared during a sabbatical leave from the University of Illinois at Chicago partially supported by National Library of Medicine grant 5G08LM007921–03 and National Science Foundation grant SES-0451122 to Alan Schwartz. Any opinions, findings, and conclusions or recommendations expressed herein are those of the authors and do not necessarily reflect the views of the National Science Foundation or National Library of Medicine.

Part I

Goals of medical care

Goals and objectives

Introduction

Mrs. M., 54, has been your patient for 15 years, and in that time she's been largely healthy. You've seen her through a broken wrist and one hospitalization for dehydration as a result of severe gastroenteritis, as well as her annual physical examinations and routine preventative health screenings. When she presented to you with a history of coughing up blood and facial swelling, you immediately ordered a chest x-ray. The radiograph showed a mass and computed tomography of the chest the next day was strongly suggestive of small cell lung cancer with some metastasis to the mediastinal lymph nodes.

You referred Mrs. M. to a highly regarded cancer center in your area that uses a team approach. Mrs. M.'s team includes a thoracic surgeon, an oncologist, a pulmonologist, and a social worker. They discuss her condition and formulate several alternate treatment plans. They all agree, given the complexity of the situation, that Mrs. M. could reasonably decide to proceed with one of several treatments. Having come to consensus, the oncologist and social worker met with Mrs. M. to discuss the options. They carefully described four different interventions and asked her which would be her choice. They also patiently answered questions about side effects and chances of success. Mrs. M., in the end, told the team she wanted some time to think about the options. They endorsed this need and scheduled a follow-up in 10 days.

Mrs. M. went home distressed, anxious, and confused. The next day she called your office and made an appointment to see you. She wanted your guidance on the different chemotherapy protocols and on surgical resection of the primary tumor and lymph nodes involved. She has realized that she may face a considerably shorter life than she once expected.

The case of Mrs. M. presages nearly all of the facets of decision making that face primary care physicians and their patients. In most cases, Mrs. M.'s treatment team will recommend a workup for staging her disease and then recommend a treatment plan that will, in their best judgment and in light of the best available evidence, afford her the greatest length of life or the highest chance of survival 3 or 5 years later. In many cases, Mrs. M. will follow these recommendations without question, because they have been developed by highly educated and experienced physicians and may be presented as the only sensible choices. And, indeed, for someone whose aim in life is to live as long as possible, they may well be the only sensible choices.

As Mrs. M.'s physician, you want her to make good medical decisions. But what makes a good decision? When physicians are asked about the characteristics of a good decision by their patients, four are often cited:

- A good decision is one that leads to a good outcome.
- A good decision takes into account all of the relevant information known at the time and does not depend on irrelevant information.
- A good decision can be justified or defended to others.
- A good decision is arrived at through a deliberative process.
  Less obvious, but just as important, is a fifth principle:
- A good decision is consistent with the way the decision maker wants to live his or her life.
  Let's consider each of these characteristics in turn.

Decisions and outcomes

Most people have a sense that a good decision is one that leads to a good outcome. However, they are also quick to recognize that someone may make the best available decision and yet have a bad outcome through no fault of their own or that someone may make a decision for nonsensical reasons and yet, through a stroke of luck, obtain good results.

In a world without uncertainty, making a good decision would be, if not simple, at least less challenging. A good decision would be a decision that was known to lead to a good outcome. For example, a mechanic who examines a car and finds that its brake pads are worn should replace them. There is no question that improperly functioning brakes are dangerous, that worn pads reduce brake function, and that replacing the pads is the proper procedure to restore the car to full functioning. When outcomes are uncertain, however, the best we can do is say that a good decision is a decision that is likely to lead to a good outcome.

Decisions and information

An informed decision ought to be a better decision. In principle, having additional relevant information should always lead to a decision that is at least as good as the decision that would be made without the information. Similarly, avoiding irrelevant information minimizes the chance that it will inappropriately bias a decision. This requires both distinguishing relevant from irrelevant information and then selectively ignoring irrelevant information. Both have proven to be difficult in practice.

Consider a couple looking for a house to buy. Each house they visit has the current owner's furniture and decorations in it, but the furnishings are not being sold with the house. Although the buyers may recognize that they should pay closer attention to the relevant (to them) structural features of the house and ignore the irrelevant furnishings, there is an almost irresistible impact of the decorative appearance that could play a significant and unwanted role in the decision.

Managing information is a key component of improving decision making. In practice, however, determining which information is available and assessing its relevance is not always a simple matter. We return to this topic in much greater detail in Part IV.

Decisions and reasons

Few patients are completely disconnected from the influences of others. There can be great pressure to make medical decisions, particularly those involving significant trade-offs, in a way that can be justified to family and friends by means of principles, narratives, or other reasons. Using familiar and well-accepted processes for coming to a decision may serve as a justification in itself, but patients are more often called upon to justify not only how the decision was made, but also why they believe the decision will serve their goals.

For example, the word *diet* on a box of cookies may provide a person trying to lose weight with a persuasive justification for purchasing those cookies, despite the lack of a standard meaning for the term as a food label. Having bought the cookies, the perceived rationale may be strong enough that the person may go to consume them in such quantities that any benefit from fewer calories per cookie is obviated.

It is not patients alone for whom the knowledge that they can provide a justification for a decision can be an important driver of the decision. The ability of physicians to defend medical decisions to peers has obvious importance in the context of malpractice suits.

Decisions and deliberation

It is often assumed that a good decision emerges from a well-considered reasoning process that analyzes the available information and weighs the available choices carefully. Decisions should not be made under time pressure or stress. On the other hand, a burgeoning literature suggest that intuitive judgments – made without conscious deliberation – are often the basis for choice and can even be highly successful.

Even when a decision is already made, however, there can be value in examining it deliberatively. Deliberative consideration may point out that the decision depends on important background assumptions and lead the decision maker to take further action to ensure that those assumptions are met. Reconsideration may also lead to further comfort with the decision because it may highlight additional ways in which the decision serves the needs of the patient. Even when further consideration results in feelings of regret (such as the familiar phenomenon of "buyer's remorse" in real estate sales), it may serve to lessen the surprise of possible negative outcomes in the future, and thus lessen their emotional impact.

Decisions and life goals

Striving to attain goals gives purpose to life. Psychologically, goals serve as important reference points for the outcomes of decisions. Outcomes that achieve goals are often considered to be successes or gains by the decision maker, whereas outcomes that do not achieve goals are often considered failures or losses. Although decision researchers always emphasize the importance of goals in decision making, goals are rarely considered explicitly because they are unique to each decision maker, and it is often assumed that only the decision maker has good insight into his own goals. The incorporation of goals into medical decisions, although amenable to systematization, thus remains in large part an art practiced by physicians who excel in communication with patients in the clinical encounter.

Each patient may have unique goals. However, the desire to fulfill goals is common to all patients. For example:

- an author wants to complete a book
- an athlete wants to play on a championship team
- an artist struggles to complete a major work
- an engineer or architect endeavors to see a project to completion
- a politician strives to achieve higher office
- a celebrity wishes to complete memoirs
- a political activist seeks campaign reform legislation
- a patient wants to have children and raise a family
- a patient seeks the financial and social welfare of her family

Decisions that impact life expectancy clearly have important consequences for goal achievement. Some goals simply require a long time to accomplish, and early death obstructs goal achievement. Others are ongoing goals that emphasize a persistent state: to live as long as possible, to run a marathon each year, or to defend a championship chess title.

Similarly, decisions that impact quality of health can also be recast in terms of either requiring a minimal level of health to accomplish goals or the maintenance of a level of health itself as a persistent goal. The list above provides examples of the former; without adequate mental and physical functioning, it may not be possible to achieve a goal, no matter how long one's life. For examples of the latter, mobility, chronic pain, and emotional stress all affect quality of health, and the corresponding goals – to increase mobility, to eliminate pain, and to reduce emotional stress – are common to many patients.

Goals may include both discrete and ongoing achievements. Individuals seeking the financial and social welfare of their families may want to provide quality child rearing – an ongoing goal – and also to live long enough to see their child graduate from high school – a goal achieved at a discrete point in time.

Another interesting feature of goals is that, although the ability to achieve them may depend on the duration of remaining life or quality of health, the value of achieving them may not. As a result, some patients may be willing to make decisions that result in somewhat shorter life expectancy, if they will be more likely to achieve a goal, but unwilling to make decisions that result in a much shorter life expectancy if they would run out of time to achieve the goal.

It is an unfortunate error for a patient to expend effort and invest emotion in making a decision that seeks to achieve some goal only to discover that the goal achieved is relatively unimportant to them. It is sensible to seek to avoid vomiting, but for a cancer patient to avoid chemotherapy to achieve that goal may be penny wise and pound foolish. One of the most important ways a physician can aid their patients' decisions is to help them clarify the goals they hope to achieve in the decision.

Goals, objectives, and constraints

In their seminal book, *Decisions with Multiple Objectives*, Keeney and Raiffa (1976) provide a useful distinction between goals and objectives. An objective, they write, "generally indicates the 'direction' in which we should strive to do better" (p. 34), whereas a goal is "either achieved or not" (p. 34). That is, in their framework, objectives are ongoing and goals are discrete. Others use these terms somewhat differently; educators, for example, traditionally define broad goals for their teaching and then associate more specific objectives with each goal. The key conceptual distinctions – between ongoing and discrete aims and between high-level pursuits and intermediate subpursuits that are meaningful as steps on the path to a higher level pursuit – recur throughout the literature on goals and are more important than the particular terminology chosen.

Each goal held by a patient implies a set of objectives that leads to an increased likelihood of achieving the goal. For example, a patient who wishes to dance at her child's wedding has the following objectives:
- to stay alive (at least until the day after the wedding)
- to stay or become healthy (enough to be present at the wedding)
- to remain or become ambulatory (enough to dance)
- to maintain or acquire wealth (enough to travel to the wedding)
- to maintain or improve their relationship with their child and their child's partner

Goals and objectives define what patients are striving for in their decisions. On the other hand, *constraints* define how a patient is limited in his or her decisions. Some constraints are social or economic; a patient may rule out a surgery with a long recovery because he cannot afford to be away from work or because he has caretaking responsibilities for a child. Other constraints are moral, and based on what Baron and Spranca (1997) have referred to as "protected values." For example, the patient who wants to dance at his child's wedding would probably not be willing to do so at the expense of the child's health, or an important religious conviction, or if it meant driving an endangered species to extinction. More recently, a large-scale telephone survey of California parents found a subgroup who were unwilling to allow their daughters to be vaccinated against human papilloma virus owing to moral concerns about the potential effect on their daughters' sexual behavior (Constantine and Jerman, 2007).

Just as patients should understand goals and objectives clearly to ensure that their decisions are going to further their objectives, it can be important for patients to clarify their constraints, to ensure that their decisions will not violate them. It is equally important that physicians understand their patients' goals and constraints; as Dr William Cayley put it, "If we test or treat just because the treatment or test is available, but we disregard our patients' needs and goals, we are not being good doctors" (2004, p. 11).

A typology of life goals

Tim Kasser and his colleagues have developed a useful typology of life goals and a questionnaire for asking about them that they call the Aspiration Index (Kasser, 1996; Kasser and Ryan, 1993, 1996, 2001; Grouzet *et al.*, 2005). A recent version of the Aspiration Index measures the relative importance of these goal domains:

- financial success
- image
- popularity
- self-acceptance
- affiliation
- community feeling
- physical health
- spirituality
- conformity
- hedonism
- safety

On the basis of interviews with patients and community members, one of the authors of this book developed a goal typology with a similar set of goals (Schwartz *et al.*, in press):

- wealth (property and financial security)
- professional achievement (career and retirement)
- family (growing one's own, or promoting achievements of family members)
- health and fitness
- education
- travel
- personal or spiritual fulfillment

Nearly all investigations of goals in medical decision making point to the particular importance of family goals. Patients who have significant family goals, such as attending their child's wedding or being present at a grandchild's birth, are likely to strongly avoid medical options that may limit their ability to achieve the goal and strongly favor options that preserve this ability. These decisions may come at the cost of their long-term health but can reflect a consistent, rational decision to sacrifice other opportunities to participate more fully in their family life.

Clarifying life goals

Goal typologies provide a useful mechanism for helping patients to clarify their goals. In a consultation to introduce significant medical decisions, a typology can be used as a checklist to catalog the patient's individual goals and to avoid overlooking any important goals. In the goal clarification exercise, it is best to keep the focus on goals, and not on the medical decisions themselves, which are only a means to the achievement of the goals.

One way to do this might be to actually ask the patient to complete Kasser's Aspiration Index or a similar questionnaire and then look at the scores. Another approach, which is both more time consuming and more rewarding, is to discuss goals directly with the patient. For example, here's how a goal clarification exercise with Mrs. M. might proceed:

Doctor: Before we get into details about different treatment options, I'd like to ask you about some of your goals, because when we're considering your treatment, we should do it with your goals in mind. So, let's think about what's important to you, what you want to achieve in life, ok?

Mrs. M.: OK. I know I don't want to die young.

Doctor: You want to live as long as possible?

Mrs. M.: Well, yes, but not if it's just surviving, if you know what I mean. I want to be able to do things that make life worth living.

Doctor: So if you could stay healthy, you'd live as long as possible, but you could imagine being so sick that you wouldn't want to prolong your life?

Mrs. M.: Yes. I'm not sure how sick I'd have to be though.

Doctor: That's OK, we don't have to determine everything now. I'll write down that you have a goal of living as long as possible, but with the constraint that you don't want to live if you can't do certain things, and we'll just leave what those things are blank for now, how about that?

Mrs. M.: That's fine.

Doctor: OK, let me ask you about some specific kinds of goals you might have. First, let's talk about family goals. I know you're married and you have two children. You don't plan to have any others, I take it?

Mrs. M.: [laughing] No, I'm through with that.

Doctor: Do you still need to take care of your children?

Mrs. M.: No, my son is 30 and my daughter is 27, and they're both doing fine on their own. I've got two grandchildren from my son. My daughter's not married yet; she's focusing on her job.

Doctor: So do you have any specific family goals or concerns that are important to you now?

Mrs. M.: Well, I don't want to do anything that would make me a hardship for my husband or my kids.

Doctor: So you want to be sure that your family remains financially secure and independent?

Mrs. M.: Yes, that's important to me.

Doctor: OK, I'll write that down.

Mrs. M.: And – this is related to that, I guess – I'd like to be able to keep working. I'm not ready to retire; I'd be bored.

Doctor: That's part of financial security, sure, but even if you could afford to retire today, you'd want to be able to keep working at something, to keep active?

Mrs. M.: Right . . .

When patients have supportive friends or family involved in their decision making, it can be helpful to suggest that patients discuss their goals with them. Supports can serve as advocates for patients' goals and can help patients check their decisions against their goals.

Using goals in decisions

One useful tool for incorporating goals into decisions is to provide the patient with details about her alternatives and ask her to build a table of goals and alternatives (Table 1.1). Constraints can also be included as goals; in this case, the patient is pointing out that she has important values that would prevent her from making some kinds of choices. The patient should then fill in the table, showing how each alternative would or would not lead to achieving each goal (Table 1.2).

Table 1.1 Goals and alternatives

Alternative	Goal 1: Live as long as possible	Goal 2: Be able to keep working	Goal 3: Keep my family financially secure
1. Chemotherapy, surgery, chemotherapy			
2. Chemotherapy alone			
3. No treatment			

Table 1.2 Goals and alternatives specified

Alternative	Goal 1: Live as long as possible	Goal 2: Be able to keep working	Goal 3: Keep my family financially secure
1. Chemotherapy, surgery, chemotherapy	Best chance for long-term survival, likely live ≥5 years	Will be unable to work for some months	Insurance coverage sufficient to pay for procedure, disability and life insurance coverage sufficient to provide for family
2. Chemotherapy alone	May shrink tumor, likely to live 3–5 years	Will be unable to work for some weeks	Insurance coverage sufficient to pay for procedure, disability and life insurance coverage sufficient to provide for family
3. No treatment	Worst chance, likely to live ≤2 years	Can immediately resume work until condition worsens	Insurance coverage sufficient to pay for procedure, disability and life insurance coverage sufficient to provide for family

The patient should discuss the table with her physician, who should point out any assumptions that are medically untenable (e.g., the patient may have misunderstood or overestimated her life expectancy without treatment).

At this point, the patient can use the table as a simple decision aid; it makes explicit the trade-offs that she must consider when choosing between alternatives. If, as in goal 3 in the example above, every alternative fulfills one of the goals equally well, the patient should be directed to focus attention on the other goals by crossing out that goal column. If the patient has strong constraints on

Table 1.3 Goals and best/worst outcomes table for swing weighting

	Goal 1: Live as long as possible	Goal 2: Be able to keep working	Goal 3: Keep my family financially secure
Best outcome	Best chance for long-term survival, likely to live ≥5 years	Can immediately resume work until condition worsens	Insurance coverage sufficient to pay for procedure, disability and life insurance coverage sufficient to provide for family
Worst outcome	Worst chance, likely to live ≤2 years	Will be unable to work for some months	Insurance coverage sufficient to pay for procedure, disability and life insurance coverage sufficient to provide for family

her decisions, she will want to focus on those alternatives that do not violate a constraint by crossing out those alternative rows that do.

Inevitably, trade-offs will emerge. Some alternatives will be more likely to achieve some goals and other alternatives more likely to achieve other goals. For example, if the patient is a composer working on her magnum opus, choosing between Alternatives 1 and 2 may be quite difficult, as the ability to work long enough to complete the piece may weigh heavily against taking an alternative that will extend life but delay completion of the piece.

The patient may well be comfortable resolving the trade-off with no further analysis of the decision at this point, particularly if the goals or alternatives are few or the range of differences in goal achievement across alternatives is small. Patients with more complex situations may need to gain more clarity on the relative importance of each of their goals. One of the best procedures developed for ranking goals by importance is called "swing weighting" (Von Winterfeldt and Edwards, 1986) and proceeds like this:

1. For each goal, write down the best and worst possible level of achievement within the set of alternatives available (Table 1.3).
2. The patient then imagines that they are going to suffer the worst outcome on all of their goals (in this example, live no more than two years, be unable to work for some months, and have sufficient insurance to keep family secure).
3. Ask the patient to imagine that he or she can choose only one goal and the outcome on that goal will be changed from worst to best. For example, if goal 1 is chosen, they would have five or more years of survival, be unable to work for some months, and have sufficient insurance to keep family secure.

Which goal would the patient choose to swing from worst to best? This goal is marked as the patient's most important goal.

4. The process is then repeated for each remaining goal. For example, if goal 1 was chosen as most important, the patient would then consider whether swinging goal 2 or goal 3 from worst to best would be preferable, and this would determine the next most important goal.

The swing weighting process requires a bit of explanation, but is preferable to simply asking patients to list their goals in order of importance, because it explicitly considers the likely range of goal achievement. For example, even if the financial security of the patient's family was her most important aim in principle, the swing weighting procedure reveals that it should receive the least consideration in this decision, because the choice of alternatives won't meaningfully influence the financial security objective.

Such simple tables only scratch the surface of decision making, but the evaluation of alternatives on the basis of goals is a critically important component of any decision. In keeping with the Voltaire's dictate that "the perfect is the enemy of the good" (Voltaire, 1772), patients should be encouraged to take manageable steps toward clarifying and prioritizing their goals.

Summary

Good decisions are characterized first and foremost by good decision process – approaches designed to increase the likelihood and degree to which important goals are achieved. Physicians can help their patients to make better decisions by helping their patients clarify their goals and objectives, and by pointing out the impact that medical choices will have on their goals.

Questions for clinical practice

- How deeply has my patient considered his/her goals?
- What does my patient want out of his/her life? What's important?
- How will treatment options impact my patient's ability to achieve his/her goals?
- Are there things my patient simply won't do, out of strongly held conviction?

Part II

Valuing health

Components of health

Introduction

Mr. D., a 55-year-old patient with diabetes, faces choices about how intensively to manage his disease. To make these decisions, he needs to better understand the health states that may face him in the future. These include states in which his blood sugars are controlled by diet and exercise alone, those in which oral agents are also required, those in which injections are also required, and those which include complications such as neuropathy, retinopathy, nephropathy, gastrointestinal motility problems, and erectile dysfunction.

Until his diagnosis, Mr. D. didn't think much about health – most of the time he just felt fine. Now the need to make these choices has forced him to think harder. Each of the health states he might face is complex and multifaceted, and he's having some difficulty in understanding them. He turns to you for guidance.

Most health outcomes involve several different dimensions of health. Moreover, not all dimensions are equally important. Here we encounter a basic paradox of medical judgment: although only patients can truly know how much importance to give to each dimension of health, their experience is nearly always more limited than that of their physicians, who may have treated scores or hundreds of patients with similar conditions and seen the results of their decisions. This chapter discusses health dimensions and subdimensions that are commonly used to measure quality of life, and introduces processes for patients and physicians to identify the importance of health dimensions and evaluate the likely range of outcomes on each dimension.

Techniques that emphasize decomposing a health state into dimensions for evaluation are referred to as *decompositional* approaches to evaluation. In contrast, Chapter 3 discusses *holistic* approaches, in which the health state is considered as a unitary entity, without explicit decomposition.

Dimensions of health

Most people don't spend a lot of time thinking about the meaning of health. For many, health is taken for granted, and noticed only in its absence – when they are ill or injured. In effect, health is "freedom from illness." For others, being healthy represents a set of lifestyle choices, often centered around diet and exercise. For some, health is a set of normal results on screening tests for markers of risk, like blood pressure and lipid levels. Health is at once all of these things, and yet more than any of them.

Health is, at heart, a multidimensional concept. Some of the key dimensions of health are life expectancy, functional status, mental well-being, social well-being, and (health-related) quality of life.

Life expectancy

Life expectancy is one of the simplest health dimensions and has historically been the most commonly used single measure of health. For example, survival durations are a common prognostic indicator for incurable diseases like cancer.

All other things being equal, it is nearly always better to live a longer life than a shorter one. There are, of course, some exceptions. The phenomenon of *maximum endurable time* occurs when patients indicate they can tolerate no more than a particular time in an undesirable health state, beyond which each additional increment of time decreases their overall utility (Sutherland *et al.* 1982; Dolan 1996; Miyamoto *et al.* 1998; Stalmeier *et al.* 2001; Dolan and Stalmeier 2003). Such patients may seek to end their own lives, or may refrain from doing so for ethical reasons or to achieve a goal that requires their continued existence. For example, Miyamoto *et al.* (1998) relate an instance of a patient who regarded his health state as almost intolerable, but who wanted to live at least five more years to see his son graduate from high school. Patients suffering from depression may be particularly subject to this phenomenon.

Functional status

Another important component of health is the degree to which a patient is capable of pursuing their typical daily activities. The degree to which pain, fatigue, and other medical complaints limit functioning is an important indicator of their impact on the patient's life.

Experts in aging, disability, and rehabilitation, who frequently work with patients facing more severe functional impairments, often classify functional status in terms of basic and instrumental activities of daily living (ADL; Katz, Ford *et al.* 1963). Basic ADLs include the degree of ease with which people can do such activities as:

- feed themselves
- bathe themselves
- dress and groom themselves
- use the toilet themselves
- control their bladder and bowel
- transfer in and out of bed or a chair

Instrumental ADLs (Lawton and Brody 1969) focus on the degree of ease with which people can perform higher level tasks such as:

- shopping
- cooking or preparing food
- talking a walk or using public transit
- making a telephone call
- taking medicines
- housekeeping
- laundry
- managing money

Functional status can be measured objectively, but selecting the functions to assess can be a highly subjective and individualistic choice. Patients who have high functioning on the standard basic and instrumental ADLs often evaluate their health with reference to fitness activities or functional capabilities that go well beyond the minima. For example, a patient who lifts weights may consider the amount of weight they can bench press or leg lift to be an important measure of their functional status; a runner may seek to be capable of completing a marathon.

Mental well-being

Mental well-being represents another important dimension of health. One component of mental well-being is cognitive functioning; confusion, memory loss, and dementia are examples of impaired cognitive functioning.

A second component is emotional tone. People generally prefer to feel happy, safe, calm, and confident. Pessimism, depression, insecurity, and anxiety result in significantly reduced well-being.

Social well-being

People function in groups, and the presence or absence of positive social interactions and relationships is a dimension of health that has received some attention. In particular, social support has been found to be an important determinant of overall health, both because it is rewarding in itself and because it increases the likelihood that a patient facing difficult medical treatments will be able to persist with them (Gallant 2003; Mookadam and Arthur 2004).

Quality of life

"Health-related quality of life," as used here, refers specifically to a person's subjective impression of their life as it relates to their health. A definition that has been cited elsewhere is: "Those attributes valued by patients, including: their resultant comfort or sense of well-being; the extent to which they were able to maintain reasonable physical, emotional, and intellectual function; and the degree to which they retain their ability to participate in valued activities within the family, in the workplace, and in the community" (Wenger and Furberg 1990, p. 335).

The key element in this definition is *valued by patients*. Two people with similar levels of life expectancy, functioning, and mental and social well-being may nevertheless evaluate their quality of life differently. In part, this reflects differences in life goals, as discussed in Chapter 1.

Using the dimensions

The multiple dimensions of health provide a powerful vocabulary for patients and physicians to communicate, particularly around questions of treatment and prognosis. Providing patients with more detailed and nuanced descriptions of potential future health states may guide them in their decisions about treatments or their expectations for their future medical needs.[1] Physicians can also use health dimensions to encourage their patients to inform them about preferences and priorities in health care decision making.

Taking complete advantage of the multidimensionality of health to categorize and compare health states requires several steps. Key dimensions and the range of potential outcomes on these dimensions must be identified. In many cases, the dimensions must be prioritized or otherwise given importance ratings. Finally, the health outcomes on each dimension must be evaluated and considered in light of the importance of the dimension.

Throughout this process, the patient and the physician have complementary roles. Patients know themselves, their goals and values, and their context, better than anyone else. Their unique contribution is to communicate their values and remain true to them in selecting alternatives. Physicians have both medical knowledge and a deep experience with the decisions and outcomes of other patients, who, although never identical as individuals, may have experienced similar medical choices and outcomes from which useful generalizations can be drawn. The unique contributions of physicians are to communicate their

---

[1] At the same time, of course, providing too many details can be overwhelming. Chapter 3 considers approaches to health state evaluation that focus on health states as a whole rather than as a sum of parts.

medical knowledge to educate their patients and to use their generalized experiences to orient patients to common features of the decisions.

Identifying the relevant dimensions

For many health decisions, it is clear to the physician which dimensions of health are likely to be affected by the decision and thus relevant to the patient. For example, in the treatment of carpal tunnel syndrome, life expectancy is not a relevant dimension, whereas functional status is a highly relevant dimension on which to consider alternative treatments. In the treatment of lung cancer, on the other hand, life expectancy is highly relevant.

Quality of life holds a special place among dimensions of health. Arguably, quality of life is always a relevant dimension because it encompasses those aspects of the experience of an outcome that are personal to the patient. Even if a patient considers all of his or her alternatives equivalent in their impact on quality of life, it is only the patient who has the necessary insight to make this judgment.

For Mr. D., who has diabetes, functional status, quality of life, and life expectancy are likely to be important dimensions to consider when evaluating treatments and behaviors that may help or impede control over the disease and its progression. Because diabetes has such a wide range of potentially serious sequelae, many dimensions may come into play. In most cases, treatments focuses on improving all of the dimensions at once. In some cases, however, treatments may require a trade-off in one dimension to benefit another; foot amputation is a classic example of such a trade-off (between functional status and life expectancy, with quality-of-life impacts either way).

Identifying the range of outcomes

As discussed in Chapter 1 with reference to goals, it is generally not helpful to take positions that favor one dimension of health over another in the abstract; it is important to consider the range of possible variation in outcomes on each dimension. When a dimension has no variation at all across treatments, it is completely irrelevant to decision making (as in the example of life expectancy for carpal tunnel syndrome treatment), although it may be relevant to guiding patient expectations. For example, if hospice care and hospital care for a particular disease near the end of life does not affect life expectancy, life expectancy should not be a factor in the decision, but the patient should nevertheless understand his or her remaining life expectancy (under any choice).

Dimensions with considerable variation in outcomes across treatments are good candidates for careful thought. Their impact is likely to be noticeable. Considering each of the basic health dimensions in turn, a patient or physician can ask, "How much do the potential treatments differentially impact this dimension?"

For Mr. D., quality of life is likely to have a wide range of outcomes depending on his treatment and his preferences. For example, if he finds monitoring of his glucose levels aversive and inconvenient, his quality of life could be substantially impacted by whether he must monitor more frequently (or experience more frequent episodes of low blood sugar). His monitoring frequency might range from twice daily to seven times daily, depending on the intensity of treatment he selects. Functional status may vary significantly if more intense management strategies result in more frequent hypoglycemic episodes. Mental well-being and life expectancy are likely to vary as well, although perhaps not as much given the treatment choices he is facing at this point; if he later experiences nephropathy and faces decisions about dialysis and transplant, these dimensions are likely to take on much greater importance. Social well-being is unlikely to vary much across the range of treatments that Mr. D. is considering; they will not greatly impede his ability to function socially in most cases or change his level of social support. Unless, of course, he is a candy salesman, a chef, a sommelier, or a gourmand.

Rating the importance of health dimensions

Once the relevant dimensions and the potential outcome variation on each across alternatives have been identified, the patient can provide insight into the relative importance of the dimensions. This may take the form of a swing-weighting procedure (as discussed in Chapter 1) to put the dimensions in order, possibly followed by some rating of the relative importance of each dimension.

On the basis of the likely ranges of outcomes for each dimension, Mr. D. might prioritize quality of life as his more important dimension, followed by functional status, mental well-being, and life expectancy. As discussed, he might consider social well-being as sufficiently invariable to drop it from his evaluation; he would certainly assign it a low importance in this decision.

Combining dimension importance with dimension outcomes

The final step involves comparing or combining the outcomes of each alternative on each dimension, with greater weight being given to the more important dimensions. This can take the form of tables of the sort illustrated in Chapter 1, but substituting dimensions of health for goals. The principle is that the decision maker seeks to compare the alternatives with a single goal of choosing the one that results in the best health, but with the knowledge that "health" covers several different attributes, some of which may be in conflict.

Another common approach involves assigning numerical importance weights to dimensions and numerical values to outcomes on each dimension for each alternative and then combining the weights and values to yield a single overall health score for the outcome. The classical approach to the combination is referred to as *multiattribute utility theory* (Keeney and Raiffa 1976), and involves multiplying importance weights by dimension values and summing them up across the dimensions.[2]

For example, imagine that Mr. D. assigns an importance (on a 1–10 scale) of 5 to mental well-being, 8 to functional status, and 10 to quality of life. When Mr. D. evaluates an outcome that he rates (on a 0–100 scale) as having mental well-being of 100, functional status of 90, and quality of life of 80, the overall evaluation of the state would be $(5 \times 100) + (8 \times 90) + (10 \times 80) = 2020$. Another outcome, with mental well-being of 70, functional status of 90, and quality of life of 100, would have an overall score of $(5 \times 70) + (8 \times 90) + (10 \times 100) = 2070$ and should be preferred to the first alternative.

As this example suggests, when the goal is simply to compare health states within a decision, the scales on which importance weights and outcomes (on each dimension) are rated are arbitrary. As long as the same scales are used consistently for each health state to be evaluated, the preference order for the health states will not change.

The example also illustrates an advantage of decompositional evaluation of health states. If Mr. D. chooses the second treatment alternative, he and his physician are forewarned that it may result in lower mental well-being than other treatment choices. His physician might choose to incorporate depression screening into future visits, and Mr. D. might be specifically directed to be alert to signs of emotional distress and report them to his physician.

Measurement tools

Several methods have been developed for implementing multiattribute utility theory in practice. They differ in such details as the rating scales used for importance weights or outcome values or the methods by which such ratings are obtained or inferred. One broad class of methods involves the use of standardized quality of health questionnaires that measure different components of health and provide a scoring system for combining the component ratings into a small number of overall health scores. Another class of methods involves individualized elicitation, evaluation, and combination of dimensions. Two of the best known approaches in this group of methods, the Analytic Hierarchy Process (AHP) and the Simple Multi-Attribute Rating Technique Exploiting

---

[2] Keeney and Raiffa's (1976) approach to assigning dimension values requires difficult comparisons between pairs of options, but this is not necessary to illustrate the practice of combining importance weights and dimension values, and more recent approaches use other methods to elicit or infer dimension values.

Ranks (SMARTER), amply illustrate this approach. Any of these methods may be effectively adapted for use with patients.

Quality of health questionnaires

A variety of questionnaires have been developed to help measure dimensions of health in the general public, as well as disease-specific health states in patients. They can be classified broadly as "preference-based" and "non-preference-based" tools; the former focus on quality of life measurement, and the latter on functional status or well-being measurement. Measurement of life expectancy is usually the purview of epidemiological studies.

Preference-based indexes are created by having a representative (largely healthy) sample of the community assess utilities for a variety of attributes of other peoples' health states. Once community-based utilities have been assigned to the attributes, a patient's health-related quality of life can be computed by mapping the patient's health state in terms of the instrument's attributes. Three popular preference-based indexes are the Health Utilities Index (HUI; Feeny *et al.* 1995), the EuroQOL EQ-5D (Kind 1996), and the Quality of Well-Being scale (QWB; Kaplan *et al.* 1976). Preference-based indexes are easy for patients to do and relatively inexpensive. The HUI, EQ-5D, and QWB are generic health measurement scales; unlike disease-specific instruments, their values can be used for comparisons across different diseases and their outcomes (Patrick and Deyo 1989); on the other hand, they may not be as sensitive to small changes in health associated with particular diseases.

Generic health measurement scales can, of course, also be used within a particular disease. For example, a 2004 study reported that HUI scores were lower for individuals who had had diabetes for a longer period and for those whose diabetes required management with insulin compared to diet alone. More severe cases of diabetes were reflected by lower scores on the attributes associated with ambulation, dexterity, and pain (Maddigan *et al.* 2004).

Non-preference-based indexes measure functional status. The most commonly used non-preference-based scales are forms of the Medical Outcome Study SF-36, SF-12, and SF-8 (Ware and Sherbourne 1992; Ware *et al.* 1993; Keller *et al.* 1996; Ware *et al.* 2001) These scales are in wide use as an outcomes measure. The SF-36 and its variations are also generic instruments that can be used for different diseases. They provide eight different functional status scales (physical functioning, role–physical, bodily pain, general health, vitality, social functioning, role–emotional, and mental health), which can be combined into a physical component summary score and a mental component summary score. There are also related instruments available for children ages 5 to 18 years, including the SF-10 for children and the more extensive Child Health Questionnaire PF-50 and PF-28.

An example of the use of a non-preference-based index in diabetes was provided by Siddique *et al.* (2002). In a study of 483 patients with diabetes and 422 without, they found that SF-12 scores were similar for diabetic and nondiabetic patients when patients did not have gastrointestinal complaints, but that diabetic patients with upper GI symptoms reported significantly lower physical and mental component scores owing to early satiety and nausea. The authors concluded that the importance of monitoring gastrointestinal function in diabetics should not be overlooked.

The Beaver Dam Health Outcomes Study (Fryback *et al.* 1993) examined the relationship between these types of measures in an ongoing longitudinal cohort study that has followed over 1 300 adults. Participants in the Beaver Dam study completed the SF-36 and the QWB, among other measures. The authors reported that they could transform SF-36 scores into QWB scores with some success (Fryback *et al.* 1997). The study was conducted in a small township in a largely agricultural area of the United States with a population of whom over 99% were white, so it is unclear how well the results generalize to more diverse urban or international populations. However, Brazier *et al.* have also had some success translating SF-36 and SF-12 scores into preference-based measures, using a more representative UK sample (Brazier *et al.* 2002; Brazier and Roberts 2004).

Questionnaires offer the advantages of standardization and ease of administration. Although they provide a sufficiently rich set of dimensions to enable most patients to adequately express their perceptions of the value of health states, they do assume a "one-size-fits-all" model of dimensions. In addition, their ease of administration must be weighed against the possibility that patients completing questionnaires may give less full consideration to their own ideas of the meaning of health and values associated with components of health than they would if they undertook one of the more time-consuming procedures discussed below.

Analytic hierarchy process

The AHP (Saaty 1980; Dolan *et al.* 1989; Saaty and Vargas 2001) begins evaluating alternatives by breaking the decision goal down into a hierarchy of relevant dimensions. For example, if the goal is to best manage diabetes, the general dimensions might be maximize life expectancy, maximize functional status, and minimize treatment side effects. Dimensions may be further divided into subdimensions to form a hierarchy; for example, functional status might be subdivided into mobility and pain.

Next, each of the dimensions at a particular level of the hierarchy is compared with each other dimension at the same level with respect to how well it achieves the criterion at the level above. For example, mobility and pain are

Table 2.1 Matrix of attribute comparisons for AHP

	Life expectancy	Functional status	Minimize side effects
Life expectancy	1	1/2	5
Functional status	2	1	6
Minimize side effects	1/5	1/6	1

compared with respect to their importance on functional status, and life expectancy, functional status, and side effects are compared (in pairs) with respect to their importance on managing diabetes. These comparisons are usually based on a 1-to-9 scale, where 1 indicates equal importance, and 9 indicates that one is absolutely more important than the other. The results are represented in a matrix of the sort displayed in Table 2.1 (the fractional entries are simply the reciprocals of the entries on the other side of the main diagonal). In Table 2.1, functional status is slightly more important than life expectancy, and both life expectancy and functional status are considerably more important than minimizing side effects.

Similar tables are constructed comparing (again, by pairs) each decision alternative with each other alternative, with respect to each of the dimensions. On the basis of these tables, weights associated with each dimension and each alternative's value on each dimension are computed by a complex mathematical process and are then combined to produce an overall score for each alternative. The computations required are greatly simplified by using software designed for AHP evaluations, such as Expert Choice 11 (Expert Choice 2004).

One advantage of AHP is that it also produces a measure of judgmental consistency for the evaluations that can be used to discover judgments that may require greater thinking by the patient. For example, if life expectancy is judged to be more important than functional status, functional status is judged to be more important than side effects, and side effects are judged to be more important than life expectancy, it may indicate that the patient is confused about their preferences or misunderstands the method.

SMARTER

The SMARTER (Edwards and Barron 1994) approach to multiattribute utility evaluation is designed to simplify the difficult calculation of importance weights for health dimensions. The decision maker simply determines the *order* of importance of the dimensions using the swing weighting procedure described in Chapter 1 and then assigns a fixed set of weights to the dimensions in order.

Table 2.2 SMARTER dimension weights

	Number of dimensions							
Rank	2	3	4	5	6	7	8	9
1	.750	.611	.521	.457	.408	.370	.340	.314
2	.250	.278	.271	.257	.242	.228	.215	.203
3		.111	.146	.157	.158	.156	.152	.148
4			.063	.090	.103	.109	.111	.111
5				.040	.061	.073	.079	.083
6					.028	.044	.054	.061
7						.020	.034	.042
8							.016	.026
9								.012

Based on Table 2 from Edwards and Barron (1994).

The weights used are shown in Table 2.2.[3] For example, if the decision is based on three dimensions, functional status (most important), life expectancy (next most important), and side effects (least important), the dimensions are given weights of .611, .278, and .111, respectively.

As in other multiattribute utility methods, the overall score for an outcome is computed by multiplying the outcome's value on each dimension (often simply a rating on any convenient rating scale) by the dimension's weight and adding up the products.

Summary

Health states are multidimensional, and individuals are likely to consider some dimensions more important than others. Decompositional techniques for evaluating health states emphasize clarifying the relevant dimensions, determining their relative importance to the patient, evaluating the health state on each dimension, and then combining the per-dimension valuations with the dimension importance to yield an overall evaluation of the health state. Several techniques have been developed to facilitate this process. In many cases, however, the process of evaluation may be more important for patients than the actual method applied. A patient's careful and thorough reflection on the meaning of

[3] The SMARTER weights are technically called "rank order centroid (ROC) weights." Of all the possible distributions of weights to the ordered dimensions, the ROC weights are those that statistically have the smallest average deviations from the true (but unknown) distribution. ROC weights should not be confused with receiver operating characteristic curves (also abbreviated ROC), which are discussed in Chapter 10.

health, the importance of different dimensions of health, and the differential impact of medical decisions on health dimensions may lead him or her to a better understanding of the relationship between health and his or her other life goals and may result in greater contentment and less anxiety with decisions taken.

Questions for clinical practice

- Which dimensions of health are most important to my patient?
- How fully has my patient considered these dimensions?
- How do treatment alternatives differ in their impact on each dimension?

The overall health state

Introduction

Mr. D., your 55-year-old patient with diabetes, has more questions. He's considered several of his potential future health states by reviewing how they would impact him across several dimensions of health, but he's reluctant to limit himself to those dimensions. "What if there's something I've forgotten?" he asks, "Or what if the impact of pain is different when I'm also less mobile? Could we consider each of the health states as a whole instead?"

Chapter 2 considered health as a multidimensional construct and approaches to evaluating health states on an dimension-by-dimension basis. Another way to evaluate health states is to take a holistic approach, and consider the implications of how the health state will be experienced as a whole.

A holistic approach is natural when a decision has to be made between two sure or nearly sure things that differ primarily based on personal tastes. For example, a woman's decision to have epidural analgesia, an IV narcotic, or no analgesia during labor is likely to be made based on holistic evaluation of the expected experience. Although the holistic evaluation will surely entail an implicit consideration of several dimensions that are personally important to the woman, which might include pain, mobility, safety of the newborn, recommendations of others, and so on, she is unlikely to explicitly decompose the health states into such dimensions, assign them importance weights, and evaluate her options on a dimension-by-dimension basis.

Describing health states

Patients evaluating health states holistically need to have a good understanding of the experience of the health state. For patients evaluating their current health, this can usually be assumed, but when patients are asked to think about health states they have not experienced, an adequate description of the states becomes crucial.

One approach to providing good health state descriptions is to take advantage of knowledge about multidimensionality of health (Chapter 2) and describe health states in terms of as many dimensions as possible. For example, one might describe a state in terms of how much pain would be experienced, what activities of daily living would be impaired or need modification, how it will be experienced emotionally, and so on.

Another approach involves allowing the patient to hear from others who *are* (or have been) in the health state, either through interaction with an individual or group or through presentation of narratives, audio interviews, or video presentations by other patients. This approach has been used effectively by the Foundation for Informed Decision Making in their decision support materials; a patient making a decision about breast cancer treatment and evaluating their expected health state post-mastectomy might be better informed by hearing other women who have had mastectomies discuss their lives since the procedure.

One health state that's often important, but surprisingly difficult, to describe is *perfect health*. As discussed below, perfect health is often used as the metric against which to compare other health states. However, there is no standard definition of perfect health. Some characterize it as "the best health you can imagine anyone experiencing" or speak in terms of complete physical, mental, and emotional well-being. Perfect health is not, however, simple absence of disease. Research in holistic health evaluation has found that people treat perfect health states and merely disease-free states differently, (appropriately) ascribing lower values to disease states when compared with perfect health than when compared with being disease free (Fryback and Lawrence, 1997; King Jr, Styn, and Tsevat, 2003).

Evaluating health states

Several methods have been developed for the measurement of value or preference for health states considered holistically. The most commonly used in research and consultation for individual decision making are the rating scale, time trade-off, and standard gamble methods.[1]

Rating scales

Rating scale approaches have a long history in decision making. In medical decision making, they usually take the form of either category rating scales or visual analog scales.

---

[1] Other methods, such as contingent valuation/willingness to pay are more commonly used in making health policy decisions; these methods are discussed in Chapter 12.

Table 3.1 Rating scale utility assessment for a diabetic patient

Mr. D. is asked to think about his health with diabetes and to provide a rating on a
  scale from 0 to 100, in which 0 represents death and 100 represents perfect health.
  Mr. D. responds that he'd give his diabetes a rating of 70. His utility for diabetes by
  this method is 70.

Category rating scales are the simplest way to measure a patient's value for
a health state. The patient is simply asked to assign the health state a number,
conventionally between 0, which represents death, and 100, which represents
perfect health. For example, a patient might consider blindness to have a value
of 50. Theoretically, a state worse than death could be represented by a negative
number.[2] Table 3.1 illustrates the process for Mr. D.

A visual analog scale presents a patient with a line, anchored at one end by
"Death" and at the other by "Perfect Health," as shown in Figure 3.1. A patient
evaluating two potential health states A and B does do by marking where on
the line (and therefore on the continuum of health between death and perfect
health) the two states lie. In the figure, state A is considered by the patient to be
about halfway between death and perfect health, while state B is considerably
healthier. With the addition of the usually uncontroversial assumption that
people prefer to be healthier than less healthy, the result is an evaluation of
which health states are preferred to others and by how much. Numbers can be
assigned to a health state by measuring the distance from "Death" to the state's
mark on the line with a ruler and dividing it by the total length of the line. For
example, if the line is 3 inches (7.6 cm) long, and mark A is 1.5 inches (3.8 cm)
from Death, then state A has a value of 0.50 (1.5/3). For convenience, these
fractions are usually treated as percentages, making a scale from 0 (Death) to
100 (Perfect Health), with state A having a value of 50. Some feel that visual
analog scales are easier for patients than category ratings and are more likely to

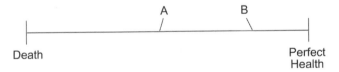

Death   Perfect
                                              Health

Figure 3.1 Visual analog scale for health states.

[2] In practice, it is often assumed that a patient who recognizes that she will spend the rest of her
life in a state worse than death will prefer death and will act on that preference. However, it is
possible that the patient will be incapable of ending her life or restrained by ethical, religious, or
other reasons from doing so. Moreover, it is possible that a patient could experience the worse-
than-death health state for a limited duration.

result in a consistent ordering of states by preference, because the states are all marked on the same line.

Rating scales are fast and easy for patients to understand; it's not surprising that they are the basis of nearly all of the decompositional approaches and indexes of health discussed in Chapter 2. Visual analog scales are also an excellent way to help a patient describe the *order* of her or his preferences for different health states. Unfortunately, the rating scale values themselves can be hard to interpret for several reasons.

First, the rating scale is arbitrary. When a patient indicates that blindness should receive a value of 50, there is no behavioral interpretation for that value – it means nothing beyond "a rating of 50."

In addition, ratings are highly context dependent. The range and spacing of the set of health states that the patient is asked to evaluate systematically affect the rating of states (but not the order of the states), particularly those that fall near the middle of the patient's ordered list of states (Parducci, 1965; Parducci and Perrett, 1971; Cooke and Mellers, 1998).

Finally, it's difficult to compare ratings across people. Although that wouldn't seem to be an important problem in an individual clinical decision, a physician who is asked to provide his experiences with how other patients consider a health state would have difficulty doing so by giving ratings without providing information on how each of the other patients he's worked with approached the rating scale.

Time trade-off

In the time trade-off method, patients are told their natural life expectancy and asked to imagine that they will spend the rest of their lives in some imperfect health state and to consider what that would be like. They are then asked to imagine that a new treatment has become available that can restore them to perfect health but will shorten their life by a given amount. Would they take the treatment (Torrance, Thomas, and Sackett, 1972)?

If the patient indicates that they would take the treatment (accept a shorter life for perfect health), the process is repeated with an even shorter length of life offered; if he indicates that he would not take the treatment (he would prefer a longer life with imperfect health), the process is repeated with a longer length of life in perfect health offered.

The repetitions continue until the patient is indifferent between the proposed shorter lifetime with perfect health and their full life with imperfect health. At that point, the duration in perfect health is divided by the duration in imperfect health, and the percentage obtained is used as the utility for the health state. That is, a health state for which a full life is considered equivalent to a life 80% as long but in perfect health is assigned a utility of 80. The complete process is illustrated for Mr. D. in Table 3.2.

Table 3.2 Time trade-off utility assessment for a diabetic patient

Mr. D. is told that his natural life expectancy is 79 years, so he can expect to live 24 more years. He is asked to imagine living 24 years with diabetes (in his current health state). He is then given a choice between 24 years with diabetes or 12 years in perfect health, followed by death.

Mr. D. prefers 24 years with diabetes. He is then offered a choice between 24 years with diabetes and 23 years in perfect health, and he prefers 23 years in perfect health. He is offered a choice between 24 years with diabetes and 20 years in perfect health, and he prefers 24 years with diabetes.

Mr. D. is offered a choice between 24 years with diabetes and 22 years in perfect health, and he is indifferent between them; he finds it very difficult to say which he would prefer. His utility for diabetes is calculated as $22/24 = 91.7$.

The time trade-off method is more time consuming than rating scales, and a bit more difficult to understand, because it involves a series of choices that require some careful consideration. It has the advantage of providing utilities that are easily understood and comparable across people, because the utility is simply the proportion of life in the better health state that a person considers equivalent to their life expectancy in the worse health state. That is, it is an inherently behavioral measure – it measures willingness to give up life-years. Moreover, it bears a superficial resemblance to the impact of many actual medical decisions, in which quality of life may be improved at the expense of length of life or vice versa.

In addition to being more cumbersome to perform, time trade-off assessments have an additional difficulty. Research suggests that some people are unwilling to trade off any amount of life because they find the idea morally repugnant. This may stem from a religious conviction that God has granted them a particular term of life and it would be sacrilegious to tamper with God's order (although most such patients are nevertheless willing to consider life-extending treatments near the end of life). In such cases, some researchers use a "two-person" variation of the time trade-off assessment in which the patient is asked to consider two similar people, one of whom will live a certain number of years in an impaired health state and the other of whom will live a shorter time in perfect health. The patient indicates which of the two people he would prefer to be (or which person he thinks will have a better life) and the iterative process continues as in the regular time trade-off assessment.

The standard gamble

In the standard gamble method, patients are asked to imagine that a new treatment (a "magic pill" in some variations) has become available that can restore

Table 3.3 Standard gamble utility assessment for a diabetic patient

Mr. D. is ask to imagine a treatment that leads to perfect health in 90% of patients and
death in 10%. Would he take the treatment?

Mr. D. prefers diabetes to the 90/10 treatment. He is then offered a choice between his
current health and a treatment with a 95% chance of perfect health and 5% chance
of death, and he prefers the treatment. He is offered a choice between his current
health and a treatment with a 93% chance of perfect health and a 7% chance of
death, and he prefers diabetes.

Mr. D. is offered a choice between his current health and a treatment with a 94%
chance of perfect health and 6% chance of death, and he is indifferent between them;
he finds it very difficult to say which he would prefer. His utility for diabetes is 94.

them to perfect health but is fatal in some patients. That is, if they take the
treatment, there is some chance that they will be restored to perfect health and
some chance that they will die, instantly and painlessly. Would they take the
treatment?

If the patient indicates that he would take the treatment (accept a risk of death
for perfect health), the process is repeated with an even greater risk of death
offered; if he indicates that he would not take the treatment (he would prefer
a certainty of life, albeit with imperfect health), the process is repeated with a
smaller risk of death offered.

The repetitions continue until the patient is indifferent between the risky
treatment and the certainty of life with imperfect health. At that point, the
probability of perfect health in the risky treatment is used as the utility for the
health state. That is, a health state for which certain life is considered equivalent to
a treatment offering an 80% chance of perfect health and a 20% chance of death is
assigned a utility of 80. The complete process is illustrated for Mr. D in Table 3.3.

Like the time trade-off, the standard gamble also produces a preference-based
behavioral value for a health state that is comparable across people. Utility is
the probability of perfect health that a patient would require in the gamble to
make him just willing (or indifferent) to take the risk. The standard gamble also
bears a superficial resemblance to some prototypical medical decisions, such as
elective surgery. In addition, by offering the patient choices between a certainty
and a risky proposition, responses to the standard gamble implicitly incorporate
the patient's risk attitude – some patients have a greater tolerance for risk than
others – and risk attitudes are likely to be important in actual medical decisions
as well (von Neumann and Morgenstern, 1953).[3]

The standard gamble has several disadvantages as well. It is both time consuming and difficult to explain to patients who are not familiar with probability.

---

[3] Risk attitude is discussed in more detail in Chapter 5.

Some patients associate the risky option with gambling and are unwilling to select it because of moral or religious convictions against gambling or against gambling with life and death (in these cases, a "two-person" variation analogous to the one described for the time trade-off assessment is often feasible).

In addition, for some health conditions, a gamble involving death seems too "high stakes" to be reasonable to patients. For example, a patient might not be willing to accept any risk of death to avoid carpal tunnel syndrome, but this should not be interpreted to mean that carpal tunnel syndrome is as good as perfect health. For such health states, some researchers use a "chained standard gamble" procedure, in which the patient first evaluates carpal tunnel syndrome against a gamble with a probability of perfect health and a probability of some health state worse than carpal tunnel syndrome but better than death (e.g., deafness). Then the patient evaluates deafness using the ordinary standard gamble (perfect health vs. death), and the utility for carpal tunnel syndrome can be computed from the responses to the pair of gambles.[4] Although the chained standard gamble produces systematically different utilities than the classical standard gamble (Stalmeier, 2002), this may not be an important concern when focusing on decision making by an individual patient.

Comparing the methods

Each of the methods has generally been found to be statistically reliable, in two senses. First, when people repeat a method with the same health state, they usually produce similar utilities or ratings; this is referred to as "intrarater reliability." Second, when people repeat an assessment a short period of time later (e.g., a week later), they usually produce similar utilities or ratings; this is referred to as "test–retest reliability." Naturally, when people repeat assessments much later, their utilities may change, because their preferences and perceptions will change over time (Froberg and Kane, 1989).

As these examples illustrate, assessing the same health state for the same patient often produces different utilities depending on the method chosen. In most cases, the rating scale methods result in lower utilities than the preference-based methods, because rating scales do not require patients to express their value behaviorally – to indicate what they would sacrifice to be relieved of a health state. In many instances, utilities assessed with the standard gamble are

---

[4] For the mathematically inclined, the utility for a health state evaluated in a chained standard gamble using deafness as the intermediate state is 1 minus the product of the probability of death and the probability of deafness at the indifference points in each gamble. For example, if the patient is indifferent between carpal tunnel syndrome and a gamble with a 30% chance of deafness (70% chance of perfect health) and is indifferent between deafness and a gamble with a 40% chance of death (60% chance of perfect health), then the utility of carpal tunnel syndrome is $1 - (0.30 \times 0.40) = 1 - 0.12 = 0.88$ (or, on a 0–100 scale, 88). Put another way, 88 is 70% of the way from a utility of 60 (deafness) to a utility of 100 (perfect health).

(slightly) higher than those assessed with the time trade-off method, probably owing to either risk aversion or the finality of the "death" outcome.

As discussed, the methods also differ in how much time is required to complete them, how difficult they are to understand, and the tools available to facilitate self-assessment by patients (Kramer *et al.*, 2005). Rating scales lend themselves naturally to self-administered pencil-and-paper surveys, whereas approaches like the standard gamble or time trade-off that involve a sequence of choices are more difficult to administer in this fashion. One increasingly common method for self-administration of such assessments involves a computer-guided set of choices. The Impact 3 Survey Generator program, for example, allows decision scientists or clinicians to develop computer-guided utility assessments using any of the techniques of this chapter (Lenert, 2007).

In the end, the choice of a method for holistic health state evaluation should be based on the needs of the clinician and the patient. When the decision demands no more than knowledge about the relative order of the patient's preferences for possible health states, rating scale methods are simple and appropriate. When a patient is capable of taking advantage of quantitative differences in preferences between the states, either the time trade-off or standard gamble may be more appropriate; the choice between them should depend on which the patient is willing to perform and which the patient finds easier or more relevant to the decision they face.

The prediction problem

A major problem in all preference or utility assessment, particularly holistic assessments that require the visualization of a health state in its entirety, is that people must often be asked to assess their preferences for health states that they have not yet experienced. That is, they must predict how they will feel about future health states that may arise as a result of their decisions.

Unfortunately, people are generally poor predictors of future experiences for several reasons.

Predictions about acute experiences

For acute states, people will experience the state for a short period, but they will experience the memory of the state for the rest of their lives, and it is the memory of the state that will be used in making future decisions. This would pose no problem if memory was always veridical, but several striking studies by Kahneman and colleagues suggest systematic biases in the memory of unpleasant experiences that can affect decision making.

In one experiment, people submersed one arm for 60 seconds in very cold (14°C, about 57°F) water, and the other arm for 90 seconds in water that was held at 14°C for 60 seconds and then gradually raised to 15°C (about 60°F – still very cold) for the last 30 seconds. The subjects did not know how long either arm had been submersed. They were then asked which of the two experiences were less unpleasant and which they would like to repeat. Of those subjects who noticed a difference between the two experiences, most preferred the *longer* immersion – more overall discomfort, but with a slightly less uncomfortable ending (Kahneman *et al.*, 1993).

In another study, patients undergoing colonoscopy provided minute-by-minute ratings of the discomfort of the procedure as they were undergoing it. After the procedure, and one month later, they provided an overall rating of discomfort. Procedures varied considerably in length (from 4 to 69 minutes), but overall ratings had no relation to the length of the procedure. Instead, ratings were related to two "snapshots" in memory: the peak discomfort the patient experienced during the procedure and the discomfort the patient experienced at the end of the procedure (Redelmeier and Kahneman, 1996). This "peak and end rule" implies that it is possible to improve such experiences as colonoscopy by *extending* them – for example, by leaving the scope inserted in the rectum "unnecessarily" for a few minutes at the end of the procedure.

In fact, Redelmeier *et al.* (2003) tested exactly that intervention in a randomized controlled trial and found that it resulted in better evaluations of the procedure and increased likelihood of repeat screening. Although few people would voluntarily agree in advance to making an uncomfortable procedure longer, this remarkable result suggests that doing so – taking advantage of the way our memory functions – could be a smart decision.

Predictions about chronic states

In a much-cited study, Brickman, Coates, and Janoff-Bulman (1978) reported measures of well-being from two groups of people: those who had newly won large sums of money in lottery jackpots and those who had newly become paraplegic as a result of car accidents. Immediately after their experiences, the two groups reported vastly different levels of well-being: the lottery winners were exuberant, and the accident victims depressed. A year later, however, the well-being of the two groups both approached that of control subjects. Two processes were responsible for this result: contrast and adaptation.

"Contrast effects" refer to the impact of our previous state on our current state. Someone who is very happy yesterday and sad today experiences the sadness more acutely than someone who was not particularly happy the day before owing to the contrast between the states. Aristotle, in *Poetics*, argues that the protagonist of a tragedy should be "one who is highly renowned and prosperous" (Butcher, 1911); the ruin of such a personage is felt more strongly due to the contrast. Lottery winners find that subsequent events in their lives, judged in comparison with the experience of winning a jackpot, lack frisson. Paraplegics, on the other hand, find that subsequent events in their lives, judged in comparison with losing their ability to walk, represent significant victories.

Adaptation is the other great force in ongoing experiences and chronic states, and people regularly underestimate the human capacity for adaptation. Our psyches seem to have a certain homeostasis about them; although the initiation of a pleasant or unpleasant experience is extremely salient and strongly felt, as the experience persists over time we soon grow accustomed to it and it carries much less influence on our daily assessment of well-being.

A regularly reported finding in large-scale studies of utilities for commonly understood disabilities is that respondents without a disability rate the utility of life with the disability significantly lower than respondents who actually live with the disability; blindness, for example, appears much worse to the sighted or newly blind than to those who have lived without sight for some time (De Wit, Busschback, and De Charro, 2000)

Several recent studies illustrate the power of adaptation. Smith *et al.* (2006) found that people with colostomies gave higher time trade-off utilities to life with a colostomy than people without colostomies. Of particular interest were a large group of subjects who had previously had colostomies that had been reversed. These subjects gave essentially identical utilities as those who had never had colostomies. This suggests that it is not merely experience with a health state that impacts valuation, but *current* experience – that is, having adapted to the health state and not to another.

Damschroder, Zikmund-Fisher, and Ubel (2005) reported an adaptation exercise that was successful in reducing the discrepancy between utilities assessed by those who had not experienced paraplegia and those who had. Their exercise asked respondents to think back on an emotionally difficult experience in the past 6 months. It then stated: "Immediately after this emotionally difficult experience, you probably felt pretty awful. But think about how you felt 6 months after the event." Subjects were then asked to make two comparisons between their current feelings about the experience and how they thought they would feel immediately after the experience. Finally, subjects were asked if they thought the experience of paraplegia would become more upsetting over time, equally upsetting, or less upsetting. Approaches of this sort that emphasize attuning patients to their own adaptation processes seem promising. Another approach that has received some attention is allowing patients to interact with others who have experienced the event they are anticipating; doing so often provides a broader focus on the event and may improve predictions of preferences for it (Sevdalis and Harvey, 2006).

Surrogate predictions

An often tempting alternative to requiring patients to accurately predict their evaluation of future health states is to have an agent who has more experience with the health states provide surrogate judgments on a patient's behalf. It would be difficult for most patients to identify friends or relatives who happen to be living in the set of health states that the patient needs to evaluate. On the other hand, clinicians who have cared for patients in all of the relevant health states are usually available. Might clinicians be capable of taking their patients' perspectives and providing surrogate measures of utility for them?

Although little research has investigated this question, the result of at least one investigation has been disappointing. Elstein *et al.* (2004) studied 120 prostate cancer patients and their physicians. Patients provided time trade-off utilities for three hypothetical future states and for their own current health; physicians provided surrogate time trade-off utilities for the hypothetical states and the patient's current health. As a group, physicians provided higher utility assessments than those provided by patients – a result that might seem promising, particularly if patients underestimate adaptation and physicians expect it. Unfortunately, however, although physicians were reasonably accurate in predicting the preference order in which patients would place the four health states, there was no correlation between the utilities provided by the patient and his or her physician within each health state.

Holistic and decompositional approaches compared

Holistic approaches have benefits and drawbacks. One major advantage of holistic evaluations is that they require many fewer judgments than decompositional approaches. Rather than requiring judgments about relevance and importance of dimensions, evaluations of states on each dimension, and combinations of dimension weights and dimension evaluations for each state, holistic evaluations take each health state as a unit. A second advantage is that decompositional approaches are dependent on the dimensions chosen as relevant; if there are other relevant dimensions that are not considered, the decomposition may not reflect the complete health state.

On the other hand, decompositional approaches may encourage deeper reflection about the underlying dimensions of the health state and may ensure that more relevant dimensions are intentionally incorporated into the evaluation than would be used in a superficial holistic evaluation. In addition, whereas decompositional approaches often require more judgments from patients, the judgments they require are often simpler to understand and faster to make.

When a decision is very important, a patient may want to try both holistic and decompositional approaches to evaluating health states. A more time-efficient hybrid procedure is to take advantage of the best of both approaches: decompose the health state into dimensions to identify key dimensions and then, with those dimensions in mind, evaluate health states holistically. For example, here's how an evaluation with Mr. D might proceed:

Doctor: One of the things that sometimes happens to people with diabetes is digestion problems. It could get hard to eat because of lack of appetite or frequently feeling nauseated. I want you to think about what that would be like so we can decide how important it would be for us to make decisions that would avoid those problems.

Mr. D.: I would think we'd always want to avoid those problems.

Doctor: You're right, but nothing comes without a cost. If we choose a very aggressive treatment to avoid those problems, the treatment might result in other problems. So we should know what different kinds of health states would be like for you so that we can make smart decisions.

Mr. D.: OK, that makes sense. So, I'm supposed to imagine what it would be like to be full and nauseous?

Doctor: Yes. In a moment I'm going to ask you about how bad that would be, but first let's be sure that you've got a good picture of the health state we're talking about – a realistic picture. I'm not trying to scare you, but I want you to make decisions based on a clear understanding. So, here are some of the things I'd like you to think about: First, your length of life. Digestion problems won't have much impact on that, as long as you get adequate nutrition.

Mr. D.: OK.

Doctor: Next, your ability to take care of yourself. Again, as long as you can get adequate nutrition so you keep up your strength, this shouldn't be affected much. The same for your mental functioning. However, your emotional well-being may be upset – it's disturbing not to be able to eat the way you used to.

Mr. D.: Yeah, and if I'm worrying about whether I'm eating enough all the time, I'd probably be pretty anxious. Food is such a regular thing that it would be an every day worry.

Doctor: Yes. Also, eating has an important social function. You may have more trouble going out to dinner or having a dinner party, if you find that you can't eat with your friends.

Mr. D.: I didn't think about that. But I suppose that I'd tell my friends about my problem, and they wouldn't mind that I'm not eating. I could carry the conversation.

Doctor: [chuckling] I believe you could, at that. Then the last thing to consider is the feeling of nausea itself and how that would impact your quality of life. Some people find nausea really horrible, but others only find it a bit unpleasant.

Mr. D.: Yeah, I used to have a kind of sensitive stomach in my 30s, so I know what it's like to be queasy a lot. My wife used to tease me that I had morning sickness. I don't care for it, but as long as it doesn't get to the point of actually heaving, I can deal with it. It's better than having a racking cough.

Doctor: OK, so think about it for a few minutes and let me know when you've got a pretty good picture now of what these digestion problems might be like for you.

Mr. D.: OK, I'm ready. It wouldn't be fun, but it's not the end of the world. Maybe 7 on a scale from 1 to 10?

Doctor: Great. Let me try to get that a little more specific about what it would be worth to be rid of those problems. Imagine that you were going to have those problems for the rest of your life – I'm a great doctor and you're a great patient, so let's say that's 35 more years. So you're looking at 35 years with nausea and loss of appetite. Now imagine there's a new treatment developed that takes away that problem and leaves you in perfect health for the rest of your life. But it's hard on your system, and you won't live as long – you'll only live 34 years. Would you take that treatment?

Mr. D.: Hmm. That's a hard choice. But I think I'd go for it – 35 years is a long time to be nauseous.

Doctor: OK. What if the treatment worked but shortened your life to only 20 more years?

Mr. D.: No way, then. Give up 14 years?

Doctor: OK. What's the shortest life in perfect health that you'd accept to relieve yourself of these digestion problems?

Mr. D.: Well, not more than two years, that's for sure. Yeah, that's about right.

Doctor: So if your life would be shortened more than two years, you'd go ahead and accept the nausea, but if you could get rid of it and still live at least 33 years of the 35 you expect, that would be OK?

Mr. D.: Right.

(Doctor notes that Mr. D.'s time trade-off utility for life with digestion problems is 33/35, or 0.94 . . .)

Summary

Health states can be evaluated in their entirety, as a whole. Several techniques have been developed for holistic evaluation, each with strengths and weaknesses. All, however, rely on providing an adequate description of the health state to enable the patient to accurately predict how he will be impacted by it, and this has proven to be more difficult than it would first appear. For important decisions, there are benefits to both holistic and decompositional evaluation of the relevant health states.

Questions for clinical practice

- How can my patient best understand an overall health state?
- How can I help my patient to anticipate what a future health state may be like?
- When do I need to measure or compare utilities for overall health states, and how should I do it?

Quality and quantity

Introduction

Mrs. K., 65, has degenerative osteoarthritis in her knee. Although her arthritis may not threaten her life, it certainly causes her pain and, as time goes on, is likely to increasingly limit her mobility; in short, her quality of life is likely to suffer in the long run. She is considering total knee replacement (TKR) surgery, a procedure with a high rate of success in improving pain and mobility for patients in her condition, but that involves months-long rehabilitation that will be more difficult and painful than her current state.

Mrs. K.'s decision is typical of a large group of decisions that feature trade-offs between future quality and quantity of life, particularly over the natural history of a degenerative disease. How should she think about her future quality of life and consider the course of her health over her lifetime?

Health profiles

Health quality, however measured, varies naturally over the course of a lifetime. Most people are relatively healthy throughout their childhood and early adulthood, with chronic illness or other deterioration of function beginning in middle age and continuing until death. Figure 4.1 depicts a health profile over the course of a lifetime. Age is plotted on the x-axis, and for each age, the subject's health quality, on a scale of 0 to 100, can be read off the y-axis. This figure shows a typical health profile of a person who spends most of his life in good health, experiencing one significant episode of acute illness in his 60s (perhaps a serious injury or a minor stroke) followed by complete recovery, and then gradual decrease in health quality (perhaps owing to arthritis) until his death at 83.

In Mrs. K.'s decision about knee replacement, she faces one of several possible health profiles going forward, depending on her treatment choice and outcome. If she chooses to undergo TKR, she can expect a fairly long rehabilitation period

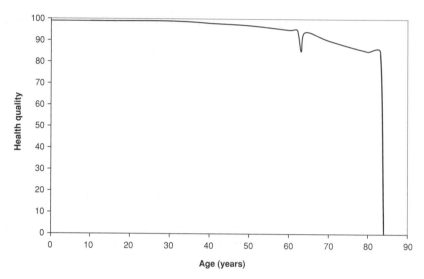

Figure 4.1 A typical health profile.

with considerably decreased functionality (and hence low health quality), followed by a return to relatively good, pain-free functioning. If she chooses not to undergo TKR, she can expect progressive degeneration of the joint, continued and worsening pain, and eventually considerable loss of function. Figure 4.2 illustrates the two profiles.

Although health profiles are usually experienced as ongoing and continuous changing in our health, it is often useful to consider them more discretely, as a sequence of health states with fixed qualities that will be experienced, as illustrated in Figure 4.3 for Mrs. K. after TKR surgery. In the pictured example, Mrs. K. passes through five health states: the presurgery state (in which her mobility is impaired by her arthritis), surgery and recovery, and then three postrecovery states involving gradually diminishing health before death. The quality weights associated with each state might be derived from utility assessments performed on Mrs. K., or from utility estimates measured in a representative community of similar women who have (or have not) undergone surgery.

Short-term and long-term outcomes

Health states vary in their duration; some health states are temporary and short lived, like the pain of a vaccination or the discomfort of a cold. Others are lifelong conditions, such as the loss of a leg or chronic disease states. Many, of course, fall somewhere between these extremes, such as injuries or acute illnesses (e.g., myocardial infarctions) that include long rehabilitation states.

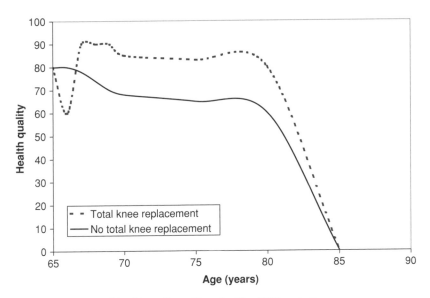

Figure 4.2 Anticipated health profiles with and without TKR surgery.

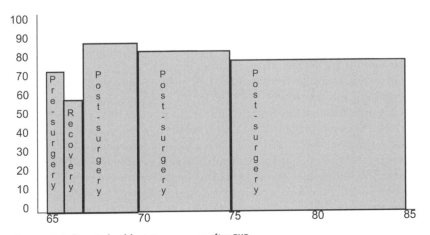

Figure 4.3 A discrete health state sequence after TKR.

If the impact of a health state depends on both its quality and its duration, short-term health states should be given little weight in decision making compared with longer term states. For example, a colonoscopy may entail two or three days of unpleasantness and discomfort; undetected colon cancer may result in months or years of diminished health. Any rational decision maker ought to give the short-term discomfort of a once-per-decade colonoscopy (or an annual flu shot) very little weight.

Although short-term health states that resolve should receive little weight in medical decisions of themselves, they may have longer term ramifications that must be considered. People live *in* these states for a short period, but live with the *memory* of the state for a considerably longer period, perhaps the rest of their lives. Accordingly, these memories may be long-term outcomes that should be considered in decision making. If memories are a complete and accurate representation of our experiences, our memory of the event should be quite similar to our evaluation of the event as it occurs (or our anticipation of the experience). As discussed in Chapter 3, however, judgments are not usually based on an exact record of an experience (recall the discomfort reported and remembered by colonoscopy patients). As a result, it is difficult to include the long-term memory of short-term states in quality-of-life evaluations.

Discounting

In practice, of course, many people find excuses to avoid colonoscopies and flu shots. In part, this is because the discomfort of the procedures is experienced immediately and with certainty, whereas the harms they seek to prevent are experienced in the future, if at all.

Is health that we will experience in the future as important as health that we will experience today? At first blush, it would seem that it well might be. The experience of three months of regular migraines would be unpleasant whether those months began today, next year, or in 15 years.

On the other hand, given a choice between migraines now and migraines later, most people would probably seek to defer the migraines, and there are some good reasons to do so. The future is inherently uncertain, and it is possible that we might die within 15 years, and thus avoid the migraines entirely. Moreover, by preserving your health now, you can take immediate advantage of it in pursuit of your goals; you can't be sure that you'll be able to do so as effectively in the future. This is the same rationale for paying interest on certificates of deposits – $1000 you can use now is more valuable than $1000 you can only use a year from now, and if you are giving up the use of your money for a period, you expect to be compensated (with interest).

Of course, it might be more unpleasant to experience three months of migraines 15 years hence, if your general health is getting worse; adding migraines to already poor health might result in a much more miserable experience than migraines alones. But now we're comparing apples to oranges; we aren't comparing the value of the migraine state itself.

Discounting future health interacts with health state duration; although long-term states should receive much more attention than short-term states, the relationship is not linear. A poor health state that starts today and lasts a year is not quite 12 times worse than a health state that starts today and lasts a month, because the subsequent 11 months are experienced in the future, and at a (in this case, small) discount.

Decision scientists commonly make the assumption that discounting is performed at a constant rate over time, and medical decision analysts typically assume that future health is discounted by 3% or 5% per year. Although it is well-known that people do not, in fact, discount at a constant rate, the overall principle of giving future health less value than present health is usually more important in individual patient decision making than precisely specifying a mathematical discount function.

Quality-adjusted life expectancy

With an understanding of the quality and duration of relevant health states, the life expectancy of the decision maker, and the appropriate degree of discounting for future health, we now have all the components necessary to develop an evaluation of a lifetime health profile.

For each year (or month, or day) of the patient's life, add up the quality associated with the state of health she will experience that year, discounted by her health discount rate (or some reasonable rate, say, 3% annually) if the state will be experienced in the future. The resulting number is the patient's quality-adjusted life expectancy. The difference in quality-adjusted life-years (QALYs; Weinstein, Fineberg, and Elstein, 1980) between the two treatment options is a measure of the benefit of one treatment over another.

For example, if Mrs. K. undergoes TKR, her life expectancy is 20 years, and her quality-adjusted life expectancy might be 15 discounted QALYs. If Mrs. K. does not undergo TKR, her life expectancy remains 20 years, but her quality-adjusted life expectancy might be only 12.5 discounted QALYs. For Mrs. K., choosing TKR provides her with an additional 2.5 (expected) QALYs, because she will experience 6 months with lower health-related quality of life but then $19\frac{1}{2}$ years of higher health-related quality of life. If she could choose from several different treatment options, she would do well to select the option that maximized the number of additional expected QALYs she could gain.

QALYs count

Measuring the effects of treatments in terms of QALYs is very useful, because QALYs provide a single measure of effectiveness that can be compared across a variety of treatments for diverse health problems. This is particularly useful when making decisions that offer trade-offs between length and quality of life. For example, when new drugs are developed that provide effective cures for long-term problems that primarily diminish quality of life (such as incontinence, hot flashes, or pain), they often have (rare) adverse events that lead to an average decrease in life expectancy. Characterizing these treatments in terms of the number of QALYs (or months or days) that they add or subtract from a patient's life can clarify their impact.

Interventions that improve both length of life and quality of life are particularly valuable in the QALY framework. As a patient's quality of life improves, the benefit of extending his or her life increases; similarly, as a patient's life expectancy improves, the benefit of improving his or her quality of life increases. Regular exercise and adequate nutrition, for example, improve both life quality and life expectancy and thus have large benefits in QALYs.

Problems with QALYs

Although QALYs provide a useful model for the impact of treatments on patients' lives, they necessarily involve simplification of how a health profile will be experienced. QALYs do not incorporate any information (beyond simple discounting) about the sequence of health states that will occur, and the degree to which a health state's impact on quality of life may depend on which earlier states have been experienced. For example, a treatment that results in a series of health states that is initially quite poor and gradually improves may provide a patient with the same number of additional QALYs as a treatment that results in a series of health states that is initially good and gradually worsens, but the former might be much preferred by patients (who are likely to adapt to poor health and regard each improvement as a noticeable gain in quality).

Alternative measures of the impact of a sequence of health states that can be sensitive to ordering of states have been suggested. Most notable among these are healthy-year equivalents (HYE), initially proposed by Mehrez and Gafni (1989). HYEs are to QALYs as holistic health evaluations, like time tradeoff, are to decompositional evaluations. The HYE of a sequence of health states is the length of time in perfect health that would be equally preferred to the sequence by the decision maker. However, although HYEs may be able to capture individual preferences that QALYs cannot, measuring HYEs for this purposes requires the decision maker to evaluate every potential health sequence, which is usually too time consuming to be worthwhile (Johannesson, 1995).

QALYs also present challenges when used to make public policy decisions. We will return to these issues in Chapters 12 and 13.

Markov models

Decision scientists formalize the evaluation of ongoing health profiles, particularly in chronic health states, through the use of Markov models (Sonnenberg and Beck, 1993). A Markov model is a set of health states (and associated utilities) together with information about how likely it is that a patient will move

Table 4.1 A simple Markov model table

		Probability of transition within a year to . . .			
State	Utility (100 = perfect health)	Mild symptoms	Moderate symptoms	Severe symptoms	Death
Mild symptoms	70	0.80	0.15	0.03	0.02
Moderate symptoms	60	0.24	0.50	0.24	0.02
Severe symptoms	54	0	0.24	0.74	0.02
Death	0	0	0	0	1

from one state to another in a given period of time (these are called "transition rates"). The key property of a Markov model is that there is no "memory"; the rate of transition between states depends only on the current health state and not the history of health.

For example, a (simplified) Markov model of knee osteoarthritis (without knee replacement surgery) might include such states as "mild symptoms," "moderate symptoms," "severe symptoms," and "death" (from background mortality), with utilities and transition rates shown in Table 4.1.

Such a model might represent the natural history of knee osteoarthritis under the current standard of care.

You can visualize this Markov model by imagining a large group of patients, say 100 000, newly diagnosed with osteoarthritis of the knee on the basis of mild symptoms. A year later, 80% of these patients (80 000) are still having only mild symptoms, while 15% (15 000) have transitioned to moderate symptoms, 3% (3 000) have worsened to severe symptoms, and 2% (2 000) have died (from any causes).

In year two, of the 80 000 patients with mild symptoms, 80% (64 000) remain mild, 15% (12 000) become moderate, 3% (2 400) become severe, and 2% (1 600) die. At the same time, of the 15 000 patients who began the year with moderate symptoms, 24% (3 600) improve back to mild symptoms, 50% (7 500) remain moderate, 25% (3 600) worsen to severe symptoms, and 2% (300) die. Finally, also at the same time, of the 3 000 patients who began year two with severe symptoms, 24% (720) improve to moderate symptoms, 74% (2 220) remain severe, and 2% (60) die.

In total, then, at the end of year two, there are now 67 600 patients in the mild symptom state (64 000 who remained in that state and 3 600 whose moderate symptoms improved), 20 220 patients in the moderate symptom state (7 500 who remained in that state, 12 000 whose mild state worsened, and 720 whose severe state improved), 8 220 patients in the severe symptom state (2 220 who remained in that state, 3 600 who worsened from moderate symptoms, and 2 400

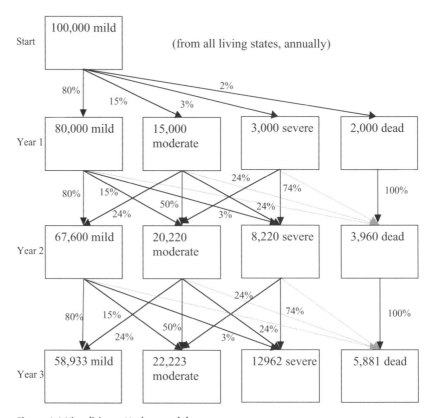

Figure 4.4 Visualizing a Markov model.

who worsened from mild symptoms), and 3 960 patients who have died in total (2 000 from year 1 and 1 960 from year two).

With the help of a computer (or considerable free time), you can continue this process until all of the patients reach the death state (from which there is no return). Figure 4.1 shows the process carried out to year three.

Now consider a single patient with mild symptoms of knee osteoarthritis. If they spend 5 years in that state, they accrue a health-related utility of 70/100 for each year, or 3.5 QALYs. If they then spend a year in moderate symptoms, they accrue another 0.6 QALYs, for a total of 4.1 QALYs to date. A return to mild symptoms for 3 years adds 2.1 QALYs (6.2 total). Then they transition to moderate symptoms again, remaining in that state for 8 years (4.8 QALYs) before developing severe symptoms and living with that for one year (0.54 QALYs) before dying. In total, this patient will have lived 18 years, and experienced 11.54 QALYs (or an average quality of 64.1, albeit with worsening quality as their disease progresses). Discounting may also be applied.

By using a computer to simulate thousands of patients moving through the model (along with a model for background mortality), an analyst can make conclusions about the expected number (and variation) of life-years and QALYs for patients newly diagnosed with knee osteoarthritis. A similar model can be simulated using the transition probabilities and utilities associated with knee osteoarthritis that is treated with TKR surgery, and the total QALYs accrued by each option can be compared. This information may be important to patients in planning their futures; it is extremely useful when studying treatments that may act to, for example, slow the progression of symptoms.

Summary

Ongoing diseases, as well as normal aging, involve a sequence of states, each lasting for some duration and each associated with some quality of health. Patients making treatment decisions need guidance in understanding the health sequence they can expect under each of their alternatives and in giving appropriate weight to states on the basis of their duration and when they will be experienced. The QALY model provides a formal means of combining quantity of life and quality of health into a single valuation that can be used to examine complex sequences of health.

Questions for clinical practice

- How will my patients' decisions impact their quality and quantity of life?
- Are my patients giving too much weight to short-term, transitory outcomes, at the expense of their long-term health?
- How can I best illustrate the course of health that my patients can expect?

Part III

Understanding uncertainty

Embracing uncertainty

Introduction

> Mr. C., 39, consults you after a public health screening program found him
> to have a total cholesterol of 260, with an HDL level of 35. His BMI is normal
> (24.6) and he has no other risk factors for heart disease.
>
> "Am I likely to have a heart attack?" he asks. "And, I've heard there's a good
> chance that taking fish oil capsules can raise my HDL levels – how good a
> chance?"

Uncertainty makes both patients and physicians nervous but is a fundamental
feature of medicine. This chapter shows how understanding different types of
uncertainty can help to put patients at ease and guide physicians to identify
the most important questions to consider in planning a workup or treatment
program.

What is uncertainty?

It would not be extreme to suggest that uncertainty is a regular feature not
only of the practice of medicine but also of life itself. At its most basic, uncertainty reflects our inability to know anything with complete surety. As such, it
is the physician's constant companion. As one philosopher puts it, a physician's
encounter with patients must necessarily include the "possibility of diagnostic, therapeutic, prognostic, and other types of interpretive error, which then
requires developing concrete plans in the event mistakes occur" (Zaner, 2004,
p. 236).

This inability to know with certainty is usually described as a lack of knowledge, and indeed, uncertainty is colloquially associated with anxiety, doubt, and
fear. In many respects, physicians regard uncertainty as an obstacle that must
be surmounted for successful care.

On the other hand, uncertainty is also the engine of excitement, serendipity,
and hope. The quest to overcome uncertainty, even when not ultimately successful, often leads to new discoveries. When poor outcomes are merely likely,

rather than certain, a psychological space exists in which patients and physicians can face the probable energized by the possible.

If uncertainty is not a blessing, it is at least a mixed curse.

Types of uncertainty

Uncertainty appears in medical decisions in several forms. Indeed, it is probably more correct to say that each decision involves several uncertainties, although one form or another may be more important, distressing, or amenable to management. There are four basic places in which uncertainties occur in medical decisions: (1) in the world, (2) in our knowledge about the world, (3) in the structure of the decision we face, and (4) in the preferences and values that are brought to bear in making the decision. Although much of this chapter focuses primarily on the first two types of uncertainty (the latter two are dealt with in greater detail elsewhere in this book), many of the suggested approaches to communicating and managing uncertainty apply equally well to any type.

Uncertainty in the world

The most common type of uncertainty encountered in medical decisions is risk. "Risk" refers to uncertainty about the state of the world that can be precisely quantified as a probability. This is the form of uncertainty gamblers experience playing roulette: the final resting place of the ball is determined by chance, and is thus both unknown and unknowable until it's too late to change the decision. What is known, however, is the probability that the ball will land in any slot on the wheel.

Most epidemiological studies seek to quantify risk. When we speak of a 42% probability that a black male has high blood pressure or that a drug that promotes successful reduction of high blood pressure reduces probability of MI or stroke by 33%, we're speaking of risk.[1] Mr. C., your patient, is certainly interested in this kind of uncertainty.

When considering patient behavior, subjective risk – the risk as perceived by the patient – is often more important than objective risk – the best estimate of the risk from epidemiological or pathophysiological data. Patients make choices, such as whether to be vaccinated, on the basis of their subjective risk (Brewer and Hallman 2006). Thus, it is not only important to know Mr. C.'s risk of a heart attack, but to ensure that Mr. C.'s perception of that risk is accurate and leads to appropriate choices.

---

[1] Epidemiologists also distinguish prevalence (the number of cases of a disease in a given population) from incidence (the number of new cases of a diseases in a given population over a given time period). Most treatment decisions focus on outcome probabilities rather than disease or health state probabilities; the latter are the focus of diagnostic and prognostic judgments.

Unfortunately, the word *risk* itself has acquired two different meanings in decision making. It can be used, as in the preceding paragraphs, to mean "uncertainty about the state of the world that can be quantified as a probability," but it is also used to mean "the probability of a harmful event." In the former usage, the opposite of "risk" is "certainty"; in the latter, the opposite of "risk" is "benefit." Because of these multiple meanings, it's easy for patients to become confused when risk is discussed.

Uncertainty in our uncertainty

Another common type of uncertainty present in many medical decisions occurs when the state of the world is unknown and cannot be precisely quantified as a probability. Instead, one may be able to provide only a range of probabilities or a more qualitative statement that the event is likely or unlikely. In the psychological literature, this sort of uncertainty is sometimes referred to as "ambiguity"; it is also sometimes called "higher order uncertainty": not only are we uncertain about the world, but we are uncertain about our estimates. We discuss this further in Chapter 7.

Another common variation of this type of uncertainty occurs with personal lack of knowledge. When a physician considers problems outside her area of expertise or familiarity, she may have a vague idea of treatments, outcomes, and likelihoods, but without further study or consultation, she will be unable to provide precise estimates of probabilities.[2]

If you told Mr. C. that his probability of having a heart attack in the next 10 years was low, he might also want to know how sure you were about that estimate. Does it vary much among people like him? Is it based on a lot of experience with heart attacks in people like him or only a little experience?

Uncertainty in the structure of the decision

Another type of uncertainty occurs when we are uncertain how the decision itself is structured: when we do not know what the available choices are or what their possible outcomes might be. In medical decisions, this type of uncertainty is strongly asymmetrical. It is quite common in patients facing new conditions and quite uncommon in physicians treating patients for problems within their specialties (it does, of course, occur when a physician diagnoses a condition outside of her specialty and usually leads to a consultation or referral to an expert who does not face the same uncertainty).

Mr. C. has asked about fish oil capsules, but may well not be familiar with the array of pharmaceutical and lifestyle treatments that are available for managing

---

[2] Personal uncertainty among physicians is dealt with at great length and with great sensitivity in Bursztajn *et al.* (1990).

his cholesterol. He is concerned about heart attacks but may not know if there are other outcomes (positive or negative) of his cholesterol level or of the potential treatments that he should consider.

This type of uncertainty is perhaps the most easily resolved, because it merely requires determining the set of available choices and their outcomes on the basis of current medical practice and clinical research and then providing that information in a format easily comprehended by the decision maker. Approaches to the presentation of decision structure are considered in greater detail in Chapter 8.

Uncertainty in preferences and values

Finally, it is very common for patients facing new conditions to be unsure about their preferences and how they would evaluate the potential outcomes of their choices. An asymptomatic man making choices about treatment for localized prostate cancer may never have considered the impact of treatment side effects such as erectile dysfunction and incontinence, much less how he might feel about expectant management, knowing that he has untreated cancer. Mr. C. may not be sure how he feels about taking medications or supplements daily, for example. Will it be difficult to remember? Will the dosing regimen limit his ability to do other things he enjoys? Will he come to think of himself as chronically ill and what will that mean to his outlook on life?

Attitudes toward uncertainty

While uncertainty affects the outcomes of decisions, attitudes toward uncertainty affect the decision-making process itself. People may be more or less accepting of risk, and this *risk attitude* is an important factor in many decisions. Choosing an option with a lot of variability in its possible results over an option in which the results are (more) assured is a *risk-seeking* choice. For example, investments in stocks expose the investor to greater daily price fluctuations than investments in government securities, and are therefore risk seeking; such investments are made, of course, in the belief that their return will justify the increased level of risk.

Conversely, choosing the less variable option over the more variable option is a *risk-averse* choice. Investment strategies that emphasize security of principal focus on low variability investments and are thus risk averse.

It's easy to see the relevance of risk attitude in investment decisions. Although its importance in health care decisions may seem surprising, the difference has more to do with our education than with fundamental differences in the tasks. In fact, risk attitude is an inherent consideration in many medical decisions. For example, if one treatment might lead to either major improvement or minor worsening in a condition, and another might lead to either a mild improvement or no change, the first treatment is the risk-seeking choice and the second is the risk-averse choice.

Risk seeking and risk aversion are used to characterize decision makers as well as decisions. A person who tends to make risk-seeking choices is considered to have a risk-seeking attitude; one who tends to make risk-averse choices is considered to have a risk-averse attitude (a person who is not influenced by variability when making choices is called *risk neutral*).

There's no right or wrong risk attitude. Risk attitudes tend to become a problem in two cases: when a patient makes choices that conflict with his risk attitude, and when patients and physicians have wildly different risk attitudes.

In the former case, a patient to whom certainty is important might find himself uncomfortable with a choice that has a wide spread of possible outcomes. This could occur even if the chosen option is actually superior to other options, and even if the patient is aware of its superiority. The discomfort with the risk undertaken might take several forms, including increased anxiety or reduced compliance. Similarly, a patient who prefers to take risks and instead selects a more "conservative" course may feel that she is betraying her own nature or dooming herself. Physicians who are cognizant of their patients' risk attitudes can anticipate these reactions and help to counsel and prepare their patients.

Physicians who are cognizant of their own risk attitudes are also more prepared to address the second common problem with risk attitudes, differences in attitudes between patients and physicians. A physician who knows that he is likely to suggest options that are more or less risky than his patient is likely to be comfortable with can proactively address the concern during the discussion of the options.

Measuring risk attitude

Several measures of risk attitude have been developed (Harrison *et al.*, 2005). One of the most useful is the DOSPERT (Domain-Specific Risk-Taking) scale, which in its most recent version is a 30-item questionnaire that can measure risk attitude (how does the patient feel about taking risks?) or risk perception (what does the patient consider risky?) in five domains: ethical, financial, health/safety, recreational, and social (Weber, Blais, and Betz, 2002; Blais and Weber, 2006). The health/safety subscale focuses on common activities that pose a health risk, rather than measuring attitudes toward specific medical treatments (that are likely to be much less familiar to every patient). Table 5.1 displays the items for this subscale.

Risk attitudes and reference points

A consistent finding in research on risk attitudes is that many people seem to have different attitudes when outcomes are gains, relative to their current health,

Table 5.1 The DOSPERT health/safety subscale

The DOSPERT health/safety subscale (Blais and Weber, 2006)

For each of the following statements, please indicate the likelihood that you would engage in the described activity or behavior if you were to find yourself in that situation. Provide a rating from *Extremely Unlikely* to *Extremely Likely*, using the following scale:

> 1= Extremely unlikely
> 2= Moderately unlikely
> 3= Somewhat unlikely
> 4= Not sure
> 5= Somewhat likely
> 6= Moderately likely
> 7= Extremely likely

Drinking heavily at a social function.
Engaging in unprotected sex.
Driving a car without wearing a seat belt.
Riding a motorcycle without a helmet.
Sunbathing without sunscreen.
Walking home alone at night in an unsafe area of town.

[The subscale is scored by adding up the ratings assigned to each item, and ranges from 7, representing strongest risk aversion, to 42, representing strongest risk seeking.]

---

than when outcomes are losses. People typically prefer a sure gain to a gamble that offers the chance of a much larger gain, but will agree to a gamble involving a larger loss to avoid a sure loss. For example, given the choice between $100 for sure and a 50/50 chance of $0 or $200, most people opt for the sure $100; on the other hand, given the choice between losing $100 for sure or a 50/50 chance of losing $0 or $200, most people opt for the gamble that offers the hope of avoiding a loss altogether.

Indeed, even when the outcomes themselves are the same, people often make different choices when they *perceive* the situation as involving gains rather than losses. A classic illustration of this phenomenon is the "Asian disease problem" (Tversky and Kahneman, 1981), given here in its "gain" version:

Imagine that the United States is preparing for the outbreak of an unusual Asian disease, which is expected to kill 600 people. Two alternative programs to combat the disease have been proposed. Assume that the exact scientific estimates of the consequences of the programs are as follows:

If program A is adopted, 200 people will be saved.
If program B is adopted, there is a one-third probability that 600 people will be saved and a two-thirds probability that nobody will be saved.
Which of the two programs would you favor?

Most people select program A, the risk-averse choice. However, when faced with the "loss" version,

Imagine that the United States is preparing for the outbreak of an unusual Asian disease, which is expected to kill 600 people. Two alternative programs to combat the disease have been proposed. Assume that the exact scientific estimates of the consequences of the programs are as follows:

If program C is adopted, 400 people will die.

If program D is adopted, there is a one-third probability that nobody will die and a two-thirds probability that 600 people will die.

Which of the two programs would you favor?

most people select option D, the risk-seeking choice. This example is remarkable because options A and C (as well as B and D) are identical in outcome, and differ only in how the outcomes are framed: as survival or as death. Another dramatic example, reported by Levin and Gaeth (1988), is that consumers preferred the taste of beef labeled 75% lean to that of beef labeled 25% fat.

In medical care, framing effects are most important when they influence one-shot decisions. For example, informed consent documents for enrollment in clinical research trials present patients with information about the probabilities of risks and benefits from the trial; such information may be framed in terms of gains, losses, or both, and the framing can impact the likelihood that a patient may agree to enroll in a particular trial (Schwartz and Hasnain, 2002). When only one research trial is available, this single "yes or no" decision is thus quite sensitive to how the trial is described. On the other hand, when patients have the opportunity to try a series of options until one succeeds, they might reasonably arrange the sequence of options to progress from the least uncertain to the most (or vice versa) to suit their risk attitudes. In these cases, the effects of framing on each individual decision may be ameliorated by the process of considering and arranging the sequence of decisions.

Emotion and risk attitude

Recent research suggests that emotions experienced by patients may elicit particular cognitive responses – including risk perceptions and risk attitudes – that continue once the emotional experience has ended (appraisal-tendency theory; Lerner and Keltner, 2001). Fearful people tend to be pessimistic about uncertainty and risk averse; angry people tend to be optimistic and risk seeking. For example, fearful people were less likely to be unrealistically optimistic about their future health when presented with both positive and negative potential outcomes (Lench and Levine, 2005).

The impact of emotional reactions on risk attitudes and behaviors demands careful attention to the timing of communication of information and decision making. A patient who has just received bad news about his health is quite likely to be fearful or angry, and his emotional state when he considers the risks of potential future treatments may systematically bias his decisions from those he would choose without the emotional stimulus. It may be better to defer discussion of treatment until emotional reactions to diagnosis have had an opportunity to play out fully.

Ambiguity attitude

Patients may also have attitudes related to ambiguity. Many people prefer options that have well-understood and clearly specified risks (e.g., a 50% chance of success) to options that have vague or ambiguous risks (e.g., an unknown chance of success). This phenomenon has been called "ambiguity aversion" and has been demonstrated repeatedly in financial decision making, particularly when ambiguous and clear options are evaluated side by side (Camerer and Weber, 1992; Fox and Tversky, 1995). However, there has been less work on ambiguity in health care decisions, and it is equally possible that people may be attracted to options without well-defined chances of success or failure, either because such options may hold out more hope to (optimistic) patients than those with well-specified probabilities (Bier and Connell, 1994; Highhouse and Hause, 1995; Kuhn, 1997), or because of an aversion to objectively quantifying such personally meaningful experiences as health and illness.

Communicating uncertainty to patients

The study of risk communication is the study of risk perception; to design approaches for communicating uncertainty to patients, it is necessary to understand how people perceive, comprehend, and apply risk information. Four major strategies are currently used to help patients understand uncertainties: the numerical, verbal, visual, and experiential.

Numerical approaches

Perhaps the most widely used approach to communicating uncertainty about the world is providing patients with numbers – the probabilities or frequencies of possible events or outcomes. For example, a 35-year-old pregnant woman may be told that 1 in 270 such women may carry a fetus with Down's syndrome, and that performing a definitive amniocentesis may carry a 1% probability of procedure-related miscarriage.

The use of probabilities and other quantified estimates of likelihood have been especially emphasized in drug marketing and in the process of obtaining informed consent for medical treatment and clinical research. There are both ethical and medicolegal rationales for this practice. The provided probabilities accurately represent the most precise information available about the outcomes of others who undertake the treatment and ought to be an important and informative component of a new patient's decision making. From an ethical standpoint, the patient possesses as much information as possible to facilitate their decision; from a legal standpoint, the physician, investigator, or pharmaceutical manufacturer has provided warnings about potential harms that reflect a good faith effort to inform.

Numeracy

The effective use of numerical likelihood estimates to improve communication about uncertainty depends on understanding the estimates. The term *numeracy* has been coined to refer to a facility for reading and understanding numbers; the term is akin to *literacy,* a facility for reading and understanding words. Basic numeracy includes such concepts as more and less, mathematical operations like addition, and the ability to work out the underlying mathematics in simple word problems. Higher levels of numeracy include statistical thinking and operating with numbers that represent probability or frequency.

Unfortunately, research suggests that high levels of numeracy are rare in the general population (Paulos, 1988, 1991). This is not to say that people cannot be highly sophisticated consumers of numerical data with experience in certain contexts. Studies of street children have demonstrated the ability to do complex calculations efficiently in the pursuit and context of operating street businesses, despite poor performance in standardized testing contexts (Nunes, Schliemann, and Carraher, 1993). Similarly, gamblers on horse races are regularly called upon to evaluate likelihood, expressed as odds, and can do so with facility.[3]

Problems with probabilities

In the Mueller-Lyer illusion (Figure 5.1), the direction of the arrows at the ends of the lines lead to the impression that the upper line is shorter than the lower line, even when both are the same size. This impression persists even among those who have seen the illusion before and know that the two lines are equal length, because it's based on a deeply embedded heuristic in our visual processing system.[4]

---

[3] If you're not a horse race gambler, "odds" refers to a ratio of the frequency of an event occurring to the frequency of the event failing to occur. For example, a horse that is a 3:1 favorite is expected, in four races, to win three and lose one, and a gambler winning a bet with odds of 3:1 would win $1 for each $3 wagered. Of course, in a casino, an event occurring with an odds of 1:37 (such as the ball on double-zero roulette wheel landing on the number 18) will pay out less than $37 to each $1 wagered; a typical payout would be 36:1, or even $36-for-$1 (in which the casino keeps the $1 wager, so really pays 35:1).

[4] The heuristic, size constancy, operates because our visual depth processing generally assumes (correctly) that objects that present themselves on our retina with angles pointing inward are closer than objects that present themselves with angles pointing out. If two lines of the same length are inferred to be at different distances, the "farther" line must actually represent a longer object.

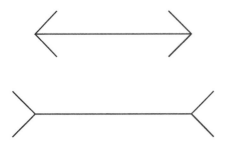

Figure 5.1 The Mueller-Lyer illusion.

Psychologists have argued that just as our visual system makes us susceptible to optical illusions like these, even when we know the correct answer, our
cognitive systems (in particular, our intuitive judgment facility) make us susceptible to certain judgmental illusions, *even when we have a good understanding
of probability* (Kahneman, Slovic, and Tversky, 1982; Peters *et al.*, 2006).

For example, consider this question from Hershberger's Inventory of Cognitive Biases in Medicine (Hershberger *et al.*, 1994):

Your patient is a young man referred to you from an inner-city screening clinic. The
patient appears to be very effeminate. Is he more likely here for a workup following a
positive screen for hypertension or HIV?

In most developed nations, the prevalence and incidence of hypertension is
vastly higher than the prevalence and incidence of HIV. This holds true even
among gay men, and equally among young, effeminate-appearing, inner-city
men who conform to one stereotype of a person at risk for HIV. Because of
the prevailing stereotype, however, this patient seems representative of a person
with HIV. And in many cases, it is reasonable to assume that the more similar a
person is to a prototypical member of a group, the more likely that they are in
the group. In fact, this assumption, which is made regularly and automatically
by the human cognitive system, is called the *representativeness heuristic*. But
as Figure 5.2 illustrates, even if more than half of men with HIV (open circle)
were like this patient, and considerably fewer than half of men with hypertension
(shaded circle) were like this patient, it would still be more likely that the patient
(striped circle) would have hypertension than HIV.

The representativeness heuristic is pervasive in estimations of likelihood and
is very commonly seen in patients' misperceptions of chance. There is a strong
feeling that luck evens out and that after a series of lucky (or unlucky) events,
the next event is more likely to be unlucky (or lucky), even when the events are
independent and equally likely. The heuristic also applies when people are asked
to generate random sequences (e.g., of coin flips): human-generated sequences
exhibit many more alternations (e.g., from heads to tails or vice versa) and many

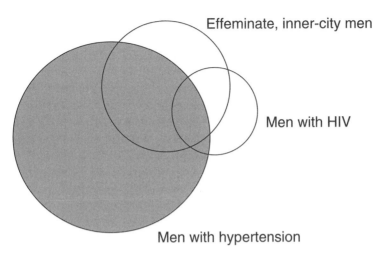

Figure 5.2 A visual example of the representativeness heuristic in judgment.

fewer long runs (e.g., sequences of all heads) than actual random sequences (Kareev, 1992).

A second important heuristic that operates in judgments of likelihood is referred to as *availability*. Simply put, events that are more easily remembered are judged to be more likely. Much of the time, this is a good rule, because events we encounter often have many opportunities to be committed to memory. One result of this heuristic is that physicians, whose judgments about the frequency of rare events are based on their available experiences (in which rare events happen rarely), may underestimate low-probability events, or they may overestimate the occurrence of a rare disease if they recently attended an educational session on the disease. Patients, whose judgments are often based on descriptions of the likelihood of events (such as those on a prescription insert or a web site) are likely to overestimate low-probability events (Hertwig *et al.*, 2004).

Sometimes an event takes on extra salience unrelated to its frequency. For example, when a celebrity personality discusses colorectal cancer on television, colonoscopy rates increase, an effect that seems attributable to increases in perceptions of colorectal cancer risk owing to an available example (Cram *et al.*, 2003).

Judgmental heuristics are generally powerful and adaptive features of the human cognitive system; they allow us to make complicated decisions under conditions of limited information with ease (Gigerenzer and Selten, 2001). When they produce biases in judgment, those biases are not limited to patients. For example, a 2006 study found that physicians were less likely to prescribe warfarin to a patient with atrial fibrillation after one of their other patients on warfarin experienced a major hemorrhage (an uncommon but highly salient and available event) than before their patient's hemorrhage. Given that evidence suggests that warfarin is already underprescribed in these patients, the availability bias may lead to significantly worse health in this population as physicians are exposed to adverse events (Choudhry *et al.*, 2006) Dr. Jerome Groopman's recent book, *How Doctors Think*, provides several illustrations of the failure of judgmental heuristics in clinical medicine (Groopman, 2007).

A good account of these heuristics is provided by support theory (Tversky and Koehler, 1994; Rottenstreich and Tversky, 1997). According to support theory, subjective estimates of the frequency or probability of an event are influenced by how detailed the description of the event is. More explicit descriptions yield higher probability estimates than compact, condensed descriptions, even when the two refer to exactly the same events (such as "probability of death due to a car accident, train accident, plane accident, or other moving vehicle accident" versus "probability of death due to a moving vehicle accident"). For physicians, support theory implies that a longer, more detailed case description increases the suspicion of a disease more than a brief abstract of the same case, even if they contain the same information about that disease (Redelmeier *et al.*, 1995; Reyna and Adam, 2003). For patients, the tendency for pharmaceutical leaflets and informed consent documents to spell out a large number of unlikely individual adverse events may lead to overestimates of the risks of the drug or procedure.

A third important class of heuristics is referred to as *valence effects* or *outcome bias*. When making judgments about likelihoods that affect their own outcome, people tend to consider positive outcomes more likely than negative outcomes. As a result, patients may overestimate their probabilities of successful treatment or improvement, even in conditions in which improvement is not to be expected at all, such as phase I clinical trials.

Physicians who are attuned to these biases, however, are well-placed to point out their operation to patients. This may be particularly important when discussing treatment uncertainties (Groopman, 2007).

Probability versus frequency

Some research suggests that people are better at reasoning about likelihoods when they are expressed as frequencies rather than as probabilities (Tversky and Kahneman, 1983; Gigerenzer and Hoffrage, 1995; Brase, 2002). For example, Gigerenzer and Hoffrage (1995) reported that 46% of university students reasoned correctly when provided with information about mammography in the frequency format shown in Table 5.2, but only 16% did so when provided with the same information in the probability format shown in the same table.

It has also been noted, however, that when a patient is told that 10 of every 1 000 people will be cured by a treatment, there is a strong tendency for the patient to believe that they will be "one of the lucky 10" and to ascribe a higher than 1% chance of cure to themselves.

Table 5.2 Frequency and probability formats from the studies of Gigerenzer and Hoffrage (1995)

Frequency format

Ten of every 1 000 women at age 40 who participate in routine screening have breast cancer.

Eight of every 10 women with breast cancer will get a positive mammography.

Ninety-five of every 990 women without breast cancer will also get a positive mammography.

Here is a new representative sample of women at age 40 who got a positive mammography in routine screening. How many of these women do you expect to actually have breast cancer? _____ out of _____

Probability format

The probability of breast cancer is 1% for women at age 40 who participate in routine screening.

If a woman has breast cancer, the probability is 80% that she will get a positive mammography.

If a woman does not have breast cancer, the probability is 9.6% that she will also get a positive mammography.

A woman in this age group had a positive mammography in a routine screening. What is the probability that she actually has breast cancer? _____ %

Risk reduction

One area in which considerable research has revealed important differences in the format used to communicate uncertainty to patients is in communicating treatment effects. If 10% of untreated patients experience an adverse health outcome, but only 4% of treated patients experience the outcome, how should the impact of the treatment be described?

Three numerical methods are commonly employed: the relative risk reduction (RRR), the absolute risk reduction (ARR), and the number needed to treat (NNT). The RRR is the difference in the proportion of untreated and treated patients who would experience the adverse outcome, *relative* to the proportion of untreated patients who would experience the adverse outcome. In our example, the RRR would be $(0.10 - 0.04)/0.10$ or 60%. Relative to the untreated patients who experience the adverse outcome, there will be 60% fewer adverse outcomes in the treated patients.

The ARR is simply the absolute difference in the proportion of untreated and treated patients who would experience the adverse outcome. In our example, the ARR would be $0.10 - 0.04$ or 6%. Out of all patients, the treatment prevents the adverse outcome in 6% of them.

The NNT is the reciprocal of the ARR. In our example, the NNT is $1/0.06 = 17$ (rounded up). For every 17 patients who receive the treatment, 1 additional patient will be spared the adverse outcome. The NNT provides a useful metric of how many patients will be treated without additional benefit for each patient who benefits; in our example, 16 treated patients won't be helped by the treatment for each patient who will be helped (who would have experienced the adverse outcome if not for the treatment). Among 16 treated patients who gain no benefit from the treatment, 1 can be expected to have an adverse outcome despite the treatment (the treatment might have helped, but didn't); the other 15 would not have had an adverse outcome even had they not been treated (the treatment was unnecessary).

The format for communicating treatment effects has a predictable impact on patients' beliefs and decision making: RRRs nearly always appear to be larger and more persuasive than ARR or NNT. A typical finding, reported by Hux and Naylor (1995), was that 88% of subjects indicated they would take a hypothetical lipid-lowering drug when informed that it would result in a 34% reduction in heart attacks (a RRR), but only 42% would do so when informed that it would result in 1.4% fewer patients having heart attacks (the equivalent ARR), and only 31% would do so when informed that 71 patients would have to be treated for 5 years to prevent one heart attack (the equivalent NNT).

Other numerical methods have been suggested, usually in attempts to incorporate additional information into the risk communication process. For example, Straus (2002) advocated the use of the "likelihood of being helped or harmed" (LHH) for a treatment, which is derived from the NNT of the treatment and the number needed to harm of the treatment (the number of patients that, if treated, would result in an additional treatment-related harmful outcome), adjusted by the patient's relative perception of the harmfulness of the disease-related adverse outcome and the treatment-related adverse outcome. The LHH is expressed in the form "10 to 1 in favor of (or against) the treatment," meaning that instituting the treatment should produce health outcomes that are 10 times better (or worse) than not doing so.[5]

Verbal approaches

A very common way of discussing uncertainty with patients relies on the everyday verbal phrases that we typically use to discuss likelihood. For example, an outcome may be described as "likely" or "doubtful," "virtually certain" or "nearly impossible." The use of verbal phrases has been studied extensively by psychologists, with two major findings (Teigen and Brun, 1999; Budescu, Karelitz, and Wallsten, 2003).

First, there is variability in the use of these phrases by people. Some people believe that an event that is "not likely" will occur less often than one that is

[5] A very similar approach was also presented by Djulbegovic *et al.* (2000).

"very improbable," while others reverse the order of these phrases. Accordingly, there is some inherent vagueness in the use of verbal probabilities.

Second, verbal probabilities are better than numerical probabilities in calling attention to the direction or implication of the uncertainty. Presenting a 5% risk of a treatment complication as "very unlikely" calls attention to the fact that the risk is low relative to other risks that the patient might face. On the other hand, presenting the same 5% risk as "small but significant" can convey the opposite implication.

Because verbal phrases are so commonly used in everyday contexts, patients are likely to be quite comfortable hearing them but will also be cognizant of their vagueness. Patients may press for more precise descriptions of uncertainties.

Visual approaches

As we've seen, numerical approaches can confuse patients and verbal approaches lack the necessary precision to make estimates of uncertainty clinically useful. As a result, many decision scientists are studying visual or graphical approaches to convey useful distinctions in a more directly comprehensible format. Two major reviews of the design of visual approaches to communicating uncertainty make several key points (Lipkus and Hollands, 1999; Ancker *et al.*, 2006).

First, some visual approaches are better at conveying information, whereas others are better at promoting changes in behavior (typically at making patients less inclined to perform a risky behavior). Second, when the goal is to convey risk information, successful graphs should display both the numerator and denominator of a risk ratio – the number of focal outcomes in the context of the total number of "at-risk" patients.

Visual representations that help patients to understand uncertainty include the icon array, depicted in Figure 5.3. In this common format, the concept of a probability of 34% is displayed by depicting 34 darkly shaded stick figures in an array of 100 total stick figures. The icon array allows patients to visually interpret frequencies based on the relative areas of the shaded figures.

Visual representations are not necessarily immediately intuitive. Graphs should always be accompanied by written instructions explaining how to interpret them.

Experiential approaches

A final approach to communicating uncertainties relies on the context provided by the patient's experiences. An example of an experiential approach is to present risk information relative to other risks the patient experiences in everyday life. For example, in 2003, the odds of accidental death as a car occupant in the

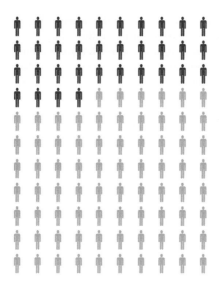

Figure 5.3 An icon array with stick figures for risk communication.

United States during the year was 1 in 18 412; the lifetime odds are 1 in 237. Many significant diseases, such as heart disease and cancer, have considerable higher odds of death; death due to complications of medical and surgical procedures is much less common (1 in 101 874 for 2003, 1 in 1 313 over a lifetime; National Safety Council, 2003).

This approach is sometimes combined with a graphical approach by arranging, on a chart, different levels of outcome probabilities with comparisons from daily life. These so-called risk ladders present some additional problems, however. The range of everyday risks used in the list and the scale on which they are depicted can have significant effects on how the focal risk is perceived (Sandman, Weinstein, and Miller, 1994).

Managing uncertainty

Most people seek to avoid what they consider "risky" – situations that offer the possibility of a harmful outcome. In many health decisions, patients cannot avoid the possibility of a harmful outcome and, in some cases, may overestimate the possibility. This misperception can result in considerable distress.

Communicating uncertainty accurately to patients is one important responsibility of physicians. In many cases, however, patients seek not only to understand the uncertainties they face but also to manage them in some fashion that will enable them either to better predict their future outcomes or to better accept the limits of their knowledge. As Zaner (2004) puts it:

Uncertainty can be reduced to some degree by having the best available information at hand and insuring that meticulous attention is given to the clinical arts: history taking, physical exams, critical use of probabilistic and modal logic, and mastery of the art of clinical listening and dialogue. It is morally imperative for the physician to understand what illness means for the patient. (p. 242)

We might add that it is equally imperative for physicians to understand what uncertainty itself means for the patient and how the physician and patient can best jointly manage their uncertainties.

Information-seeking strategies

One major strategy for managing uncertainty is seeking additional information. New information may enable a patient to reduce their uncertainty directly, as when new research studies provide more insight into patient outcomes and increase the likelihood that a particular treatment will or will not be beneficial. Even when new information does not yield greater certainty about outcomes, it may serve to narrow the range of the uncertainty.

The primary source of new clinical information is medical research. Most clinical research is explicitly motivated by a need to reduce the uncertainties around etiology, prevention, diagnosis, treatment, or prognosis. Chapter 9 considers the value of clinical research and obtaining additional information in medical decisions in some detail.

Affective strategies

Coping

One of the most pervasive findings about the perception of harmful uncertainties is that they are related to the degree to which the outcomes are dreaded, unfamiliar, and uncontrollable (Slovic *et al.*, 1981). These factors provide some guidance for patients seeking to cope with risky health decisions, particularly when the probabilities of harm are objectively small but appear large to the patient.

To the degree to which a patient's dread of a harmful outcome can be reduced, the patient may consider the outcome less likely. Dread is a characteristic of the outcome, not its likelihood. Dread can be reduced but successful interventions are individual specific. For some patients, opportunities to express their fears fully can effectively reduce dread. Some may find solace in the support of family and friends. Others may call on relaxation techniques and similar practices. Physicians can suggest that patients reflect on how they have coped with fears in other areas of their lives.

Unfamiliar outcomes are often perceived as more risky. For example, a nerve gas attack is much less familiar than a gunshot and is accordingly regarded as riskier, even if the patient knows it to be less probable. Communicating information about the outcomes themselves (as well as their probabilities) and referring patients to support groups are common ways of decreasing unfamiliarity.

Finally, uncontrollable outcomes are typically seen as riskier, and more difficult to bear, than outcomes that afford opportunities for exerting control. Although in many cases patients may be truly limited in the amount of control they can exert over their disease, the research literature has increasingly documented the impact of modifiable lifestyle factors (including diet, exercise, stress levels, mental outlook, etc.) on the progress of diseases and the efficacy of their treatment. Physicians who can offer their patients elements of control over their short- or long-term outcomes may enhance their patients' coping. When physicians do not direct patients to controllable factors, however, distressed patients may invent such factors – and methods for controlling them – themselves, and not always to their long-term benefit (e.g., see Burstein *et al.*, 1999).

Embracing hope

As difficult as it may seem, patients and physicians can, at times, actually embrace uncertainties around health care. Uncertainty may lead to dread, but it may also lead to hope.

Hope is valuable not only in itself, but also because it may lead to better medical outcomes. A recent study of pediatric transplant patients found that higher levels of hope were associated with lower levels of depression; because depression contributes to nonadherence to treatment, hope may contribute to adherence behaviors (Maikranz *et al.*, 2006). At the same time, increased uncertainty contributed to greater depression, so both uncertainty-reducing and hope-enhancing strategies may be warranted.

On the other hand, prognostic uncertainty may lead to unrealistic hopes that delay opportunities for, for example, palliative care that may better serve the patient's goals (De Graves and Aranda, 2005). Patients who can approach their possibilities in a positive way, but retain a clear-eyed view of the probabilities, are likely to achieve the greatest benefit from embracing uncertainty (Bursztajn *et al.*, 1990).

Summary

Uncertainty is a fundamental fact of medicine, and one that concerns both patients and physicians. Patients experience several types of uncertainty, and physicians have a variety of tools at their disposal for helping patients understand uncertainty and their feelings toward it, as well as techniques for reducing and managing uncertainty. The decision science literature provides evidence-based recommendations for how and when to use these tools and techniques.

Questions for clinical practice

- What are the most important uncertainties in the decision facing my patient?
- How does my patient regard risk and uncertainty in his or her life? Does she or he believe in taking chances to achieve big rewards or prefer to opt for smaller but surer results?
- How can I most effectively and accurately communicate the level of uncertainty associated with a diagnosis, a treatment, or a prognosis to my patient?
- How can I help my patient to cope with their lack of certainty about outcomes or options?

Chance and choice

Introduction

Mr. P., 67, showed an increase in his PSA level at his most recent physical. He underwent a needle biopsy of his prostate which found cancerous cells. He is now considering whether to undergo a radical prostatectomy, to have a radiation procedure, or to manage his cancer expectantly, through watchful waiting. Each treatment option offers some hope of forestalling or curtailing the growth of the cancer and permitting him to live his full life expectancy (perhaps dying with prostate cancer, rather than of it). However, each option also involves risks of serious side effects.

Most medical decisions present the possibility of several possible outcomes, with no certainty about which will actually occur. This chapter introduces tools for evaluating and comparing such options by combining information about the probabilities of outcomes with insights about the values of outcomes. As such, this chapter builds more heavily than most on the preceding chapters.

The expectation principle

The key rule for evaluating options that include outcomes that are uncertain is the expectation principle: the "expected value" of being exposed to the possibility of an outcome is determined by the value of the outcome and the frequency with which it would be experienced if you were exposed to the possibility repeatedly. For example, facing a 1-in-12 chance of losing a year of life expectancy should be evaluated as facing a certain loss of 1 month (1/12th of 1 year) of life expectancy. The expected value of such an option is loss of 1 month of life.

At the level of a population of patients, this principle is easy to understand. If 1 200 patients face the option, about 100 of them (1 in 12) will lose 1 year of life, while the other 1 100 do not. The net result is 100 years of life lost to the group of 1 200 patients or, on average, a loss of 1 month per patient.

What puts the expectation principle at odds with actual experience, however, is that no individual patient in that group ever loses a month of life; each loses either a year or nothing. But because we do not know in advance, *at the time of the decision*, whether a particular patient will be one of the lucky ones or one of the unlucky ones, each patient is in an identical state of uncertainty and faces the same expected, or average, loss of one month of life if they must face this option. Moreover, although a patient may make a particular decision only once, everyone faces a myriad of decisions throughout the course of their life. Applying the expectation principle to each individual decision maximizes the expected results of the entire sequence of life decisions.

Maximizing expected value

The expectation principle is useful when comparing treatment choices. A treatment that has an expected loss of one month of life is likely to be preferable to one that has an expected loss of one year of life.

More formally, in many cases, people who can measure a "value" related to their goals want to (and ought to) make decisions to maximize their expected value. If a patient's goal is to live as long as possible, their value is measured in life expectancy, and their choices should seek to maximize their expected length of life. For example, a 50-year-old patient who is expected to live to 70 years (e.g., based on the patient's risk factors) should agree to a procedure which offers them an 80% chance of living to 72, and a 20% chance of dying at 69, because the procedure has an expectation of 71.4 years.

Multiple outcomes

Because no treatments are completely sure, every treatment offers some probability of at least two outcomes (successful treatment and failed treatment), and most may result in other outcomes. For example, the most common long-term outcomes from radical prostatectomy might be those shown in Table 6.1.[1]

With knowledge of the probabilities and values associated with each outcome for a particular patient, the expectation principle enables us to develop a measure of the expected value of choosing this treatment by multiplying each outcome's value by its probability and adding each of these products together. Using the data in Table 6.1, for example, the value of radical prostatectomy is 88.8:

$$(100 \times 66\%) + (80 \times 20\%) + (70 \times 4\%) + (40 \times 10\%)$$
$$= 66 + 16 + 2.8 + 4 = 88.8$$

---

[1] Of course, there are more possible outcomes than these (e.g., cure with both incontinence and erectile dysfunction), but these serve to illustrate the approach.

Table 6.1 Sample long-term outcomes of radical prostatectomy

Outcome	Probability estimate (%)	Value (0–100)
Complete cure (no significant tumor reappearance or progression before death would occur of other causes)	66	100
Cure with permanent erectile dysfunction	20	80
Cure with permanent urinary incontinence	4	70
Tumor reappearance leading to early mortality	10	40

Of course, this requires that we have listed all of the relevant outcomes, and that each is exclusive of the others (the probabilities must add up to 100%).

Unfortunately, many treatment options offer a large number of outcomes, each with a small independent probability, which means that there are a potentially enormous number of combinations of outcomes that could occur. For example, an informed consent document for radical prostatectomy from the Department of Health of the Government of Western Australia (2002) lists the following potential adverse outcomes (other than those associated with anesthetics):

- deep vein thrombosis, which may lead to pulmonary embolism, and, rarely, death
- collapsed lungs, requiring physiotherapy
- wound infection, requiring antibiotics or reopening
- urinary infection, requiring antibiotics
- bleeding during surgery, requiring transfusion
- erectile dysfunction, temporary or permanent
- urinary incontinence (stress leakage common, significant incontinence rare)
- bladder scarring making urination difficult, requiring surgical intervention
- pelvic abscess, possibly requiring drainage
- rectal injury, requiring a temporary colostomy
- reappearance of the tumor

If each of these 11 outcomes has an independent probability of occurrence, there are over 2 000 different combinations of outcomes, many with miniscule probabilities.[2] Assigning probabilities and values to each of these possible results may be useful for a computerized decision model but is unlikely to be of much help to a patient.

---

[2] To be exact, 2 048 combinations. If each event can independently occur or not occur, the number of potential combinations of the 11 events is 2^{11}.

The informed consent document illustrates another challenge in applying the expectation principle. In many cases, it is difficult or impossible to obtain objective probabilities for outcomes or their combinations. When this occurs, patients should fall back on subjective probabilities (their own or, more likely, those of their physician), as discussed in Chapter 5. These subjective probabilities embody the decision maker's best estimates of the likelihood of relevant outcomes on the basis of the experience, expertise, evidence, and advice available to him at the time of the decision. Although they may not be perfectly faithful to the (unknown) objective probabilities, they represent a reasonable alternative (Edwards, 1954).

The preparation principle

The expectation principle is only useful before a decision is made. Once a patient has committed to a decision, he will experience one of its actual outcomes, not the average outcome. Consider a more extreme example: a 55-year-old patient facing a 1-in-12 chance of losing 12 years of 20-year life expectancy. This patient would not be well-served by preparing for a life shortened by one year. If he needs to get his affairs in order before he dies, he must do so under the assumption that he may only live to age 63.

This is why patients should respect fairly small probabilities of death or permanently disabling outcomes.[3] Although such chances may not greatly diminish the expected value of a treatment (and perhaps should not actually weigh against choosing the treatment), once chosen, a patient may be wise to plan ahead of the possibility of catastrophe (by preparing their will, signing an advance directive, doing things they'd always meant to do, etc.).

That is, *once a decision has been made, one must plan for the potential outcomes.* We call this the "preparation principle."

Following this principle, many patients are sensitive not only to the expected value of an option, but also to its variability, or spread. A 1-in-12 chance of losing 12 years has the same expectation as a 1-in-3 chance of losing 3 years, but a much larger spread. When options are equal in expectation, preference for spread is directly related to risk attitude, discussed in Chapter 5.

On the other hand, few medical decisions promise such precise outcomes. In practice, "losing a year of life" itself really means losing a year of life, *on average.* Some patients will lose more than a year, some less, but the spread is small enough that we are comfortable characterizing the outcome as loss of a year.

---

[3] In this context, "fairly small" means larger than the patient is exposed to regularly. If the chance of death is smaller than what they experience during their daily commute, for example, it's probably too small to trigger estate planning (or perhaps they should be making those plans before their next work week!).

Expected what?

The maximization of expected value in risky decision making has a long history.[4] The mathematics of expectation made their earliest well-known appearance in Blaise Pascal's solution to the "Problem of Points" in 1654. The Problem of Points assumes that there is a game in which the two players have an equal chance to win a point on each round of the game, and the object of the game is to be ahead by some number of points. For example, the player who leads their opponent by six points might win, and the winner gets the entire amount of money wagered on the game. The Problem itself is this: if the game is ended early, for example, with one player ahead by only three points, how should the wager be fairly split between the players? Pascal, in correspondence with his friend Pierre Fermat, worked out the idea that the each player should receive their expected value if the game were to continue from that point.

Expected value alone was not a perfect solution to the valuation of risky gambles, however. The St. Petersburg Paradox, a classic demonstration of the limitations of expected value, was described by Nicolas Bernoulli in 1713 (and later solved by his cousin Daniel Bernoulli in 1738). In the Paradox, you are offered a chance to play a simple game of coin flipping until a tail comes up. If the first flip is a tail, you win $1. If not, you keep flipping, but each time you flip a head, the jackpot doubles, until you flip a tail and are paid. The question posed by N. Bernoulli was how much would be a fair price to pay to play such a game?

The paradox arises because the expected value of the game is infinite,[5] but few are willing to pay more than a few dollars to pay. Daniel Bernoulli's resolution was to note that the pleasure or utility of money decreases as you get more of it: $10 means more to a poor person than to a rich person. As he put it: *utility resulting from any small increase in wealth will be inversely proportionate to the quantity of goods previously possessed.* As a consequence, the doubling of the jackpot's value results in less than a doubling of the jackpot's utility. Instead of computing the expected value of the game, Bernoulli argued for computing the expected utility of the game. Based on his particular theory of the relationship between value and utility, Bernoulli concluded that the game was worth $2 (Bernoulli, 1954). Bernoulli's work represents the true inception of expected utility as a guide to decision making (Mellers, 2000).

Jeremy Bentham, a moral philosopher, picked up on these ideas in his discussion of the "hedonic calculus," a system for determining the amount of pleasure or good associated with an outcome. Bentham considered the utilities of

---

[4] Those interested in the history and science of probability can learn more from Gigerenzer *et al.* (1989).

[5] Because the sum of the series $1 + (1/2)^*\$2 + (1/4)^*\$4 + (1/8)^*\$8 + \ldots$ is an infinite series of $1 + \$1 + \$1 + \ldots$

outcomes to be related to their intensity, duration, certainty, nearness, likelihood of later producing further pleasure, unlikelihood of later producing pain, and the number of individuals over which they extend[6] (Bentham, 1970).

The next important extension to expected utility theory was proposed to guide decision making in cases where perfect data about the probabilities of outcomes are not available. Subjective expected utility (SEU) theory, generally credited to Savage (1954), simply posited that where objective probabilities are not available, subjective probabilities or beliefs should be used in their stead. In the absence of other data, subjective probabilities were argued to represent the best approximation of the actual likelihood of events.

When the uncertain outcomes cease to be monetary and become, instead, health states, the maximization of expected utility translates naturally to the maximization of health-related (usually multiattribute) quality of life. An immediate difficulty in working out the expected value of a treatment arises when the possible outcomes are difficult to compare. How does one calculate the expected value of a neurosurgery that involves a 2% chance of blindness? To make these calculations, even roughly, requires a way of measuring expected quality of life, or utility; tools for doing so were discussed in the early chapters of this book.

What about a 2% chance of blindness, a 1% chance of death, and a 4% chance of chronic headaches for a year? Here we need a measure that incorporates outcomes of different durations that affect both quality of life and length of life. Chapter 4 discussed such a measure, the quality-adjusted life year (QALY), and such decisions are often analyzed with the goal of maximizing the patient's expected QALYs.

What about goals beyond simply quality and length of life? Few models exist for combining such goals into a single measure; instead, patients may have to determine which of their options maximize each of their goals and, if the options conflict, prioritize their goals.

Expectation and calculation

Calculating expected values, utilities, or QALYs involves a great deal of fairly tedious computation. The operations are quite simple: multiple probability by value, utility, or QALY and add up all the products, but there are many of them,

---

[6] Bentham's mnemonic for these attributes was a short poem:

Intense, long, certain, speedy, fruitful, pure –
Such marks in pleasures and in pains endure.
Such pleasures seek, if private be thy end:
If it be public, wide let them extend.
Such pains avoid, whichever be thy view:
If pains must come, let them extend to few.

Table 6.2 Expected utility worksheet

Outcome name	Probability		Utility/value		Probability × Utility
_____	_____	×	_____	=	_____
_____	_____	×	_____	=	_____
_____	_____	×	_____	=	_____
_____	_____	×	_____	=	_____
_____	_____	×	_____	=	_____
_____	_____	×	_____	=	_____
_____	_____	×	_____	=	_____
_____	_____	×	_____	=	_____
_____	_____	×	_____	=	_____
_____	_____	×	_____	=	_____

Sum of probabilities should be   100%
Expected utility (sum of probability × utility):

and it's easy to lose track. The simplest way to keep the calculations straight is to use a worksheet, like that shown in Table 6.2.[7]

An electronic version of the worksheet is available on the web at http://araw. mede.uic.edu/cgi-bin/ev.cgi.

What do patients really do?

Maximizing SEU is a normative strategy: it describes how patients *should* make choices to achieve the best possible outcomes (in utility terms). In contrast, descriptive theories of human decision making seek to describe, explain, and predict *actual* decision behavior.

Descriptive utility theories

Historically, maximizing SEU was also an early candidate for a descriptive theory (Edwards, 1954).[8] Between 1955 and 1980, however, a series of studies

---

[7] Because the basic operation is two-dimensional, like multiplying the length and width of a square to find its area, there are also some geometric approaches possible. For example, if probabilities and utilities are only estimated in discrete increments (e.g., 5% or 5 points on a 100-point scale), one could even represent each possible outcome by a rectangle made of colored LEGO™ bricks or similar building blocks, with length corresponding to probability and width to utility. The overall expected value would be formed by connecting all of the individual rectangles. Because the weight of such blocks is directly proportional to the area (each block is equally dense), expected values of different options can then by compared by weighing the bricks against each other.

[8] Methods designed to bring actual behavior closer to the results that could be achieved through normative solutions are referred to as "prescriptive" approaches. This book is an example.

established that people regularly make decisions that violate the principles of maximizing SEU. One important set of examples concerns the principle of "descriptive invariance": if option A is preferred to option B, it should be preferred regardless of how the two options are described (as long as the same information is presented). A key violation of descriptive invariance is illustrated by gain/loss framing effects, such as the Asian disease problem described in Chapter 5 (Tversky and Kahneman, 1981).

This phenomenon – risk aversion when outcomes are framed as gains and risk seeking when they are framed as losses – has been widely replicated, including in studies of patients and physicians around medical treatment decisions (McNeil *et al.*, 1982).[9] It implies that people don't evaluate decision outcomes in isolation but relative to their current state. That is, we evaluate the utilities of gains or losses from our current state, not the utilities of final states. It also implies diminishing marginal value (gaining or losing the next dollar is worth less and less) and loss aversion (disutility of losses is higher than utility of equivalent gains). Taken together, these phenomena imply a value function like that shown in Figure 6.1(A). The curve of the function illustrates diminishing marginal value; the steeper curve for losses illustrates loss aversion.

Another series of studies established that people regularly give too much subjective weight to low probabilities (but not to zero) and too little subjective weight to high probabilities (but not to certainty). For example, a recent study of medical decision making found that probabilities of 10% were given weights equivalent to 22%; probabilities of 90% were given weights equivalent to 68% (Bleichrodt and Pinto, 2000). This phenomenon is illustrated in Figure 6.1(B).

The best known descriptive theory of decision making that incorporates these phenomena is cumulative prospect theory (Tversky and Kahneman, 1992), but there are several other descriptive theories that predict similar behavior, albeit with slightly different mechanisms (Luce and Fishburn, 1991; Birnbaum, Patton, and Lott, 1999; Miyamoto, 2000).

The practical import of these findings is that people, unaided, will not usually make decisions that maximize SEU, particularly in cases that involve a combination of gains and losses from their current state and probabilities that are very small or very large. Because this characterizes many, if not most, significant medical decisions, there are good opportunities for physicians to alert their patients to these phenomena and to aid their patients in ensuring that their intuitive choices will in fact serve their goals.

---

[9] One recent paper found that risk attitudes for a hypothetical health decision in the domain of gains (measured in "relapse-free days") were risk neutral overall, although they varied widely among respondents. Risk attitude for losses was not measured in this study (Prosser and Wittenberg, 2007).

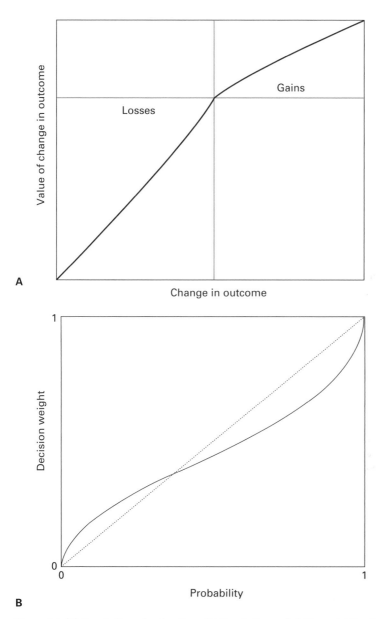

A

B

Figure 6.1 (A) Descriptive value function. (B) Descriptive probability weighting function.

Table 6.3 Sample long-term outcomes of watchful waiting

Outcome	Probability estimate (%)	Value (0–100)
No significant tumor progression before death would occur of other causes	67	100
Tumor progression leading to permanent erectile dysfunction	2	80
Tumor progression leading to permanent urinary incontinence	2	70
Tumor progression leading to early mortality	29	40

Alternatives to expectation

Multiplying values by decision weights and maximizing expected value (or utility, etc.) is not the only way that choices can be made. Although proponents of expectation can demonstrate that it is optimal (i.e., there is no other strategy that will reliably outperform it, on average, in achieving goals that can be quantified), it is data intensive, time consuming, and cognitively difficult to perform a complete, or even approximate, expected value calculation for a significant health choice such as prostatectomy. Several "biased" strategies that rely on considerably fewer data and almost no calculation have also been described and have been shown to characterize decision behavior in some cases.

Considering again Mr. P.'s decision, and using the sample long-term outcomes in Table 6.1 for prostatectomy and Table 6.3 for watchful waiting, this section illustrates four well-known nonexpectation strategies.

Lexicographic choices

A "lexicographic" strategy is one that compares options attribute by attribute, typically beginning with the most important attribute, and concluding as soon as one option clearly outperforms the other on an attribute. Because no trade-offs are made between attributes,[10] and many fewer attributes (often just one) are considered, lexicographic strategies are easy and fast. In situations in which the patient has a single primary goal that's much more important than the others, or in which performance on most attributes are correlated, the lexicographic strategy may be nearly as good as strategies based on expectation, as well.

If Mr. P.'s most important attribute is length of life (as suggested by his value ratings), a lexicographic strategy would conclude that surgery is the best choice.

---

[10] In the decision literature, strategies which proceed without the possibility of trade-offs are referred to as "noncompensatory."

Minimax

Minimax is short for "minimize the maximum loss," and that's exactly what the minimax strategy is about. People who use this strategy determine the worst case[11] that could occur under each of their options and choose the option that has the best worst case. This results in very conservative decisions. For example, given a choice between a procedure that has a 1% chance of death and a 99% chance of cure and another with a 50% chance of partial failure (making their condition somewhat worse) and a 50% chance of partial cure (making their condition somewhat better), the true minimaxer will select the latter procedure. Indeed, a pure minimax strategy will never choose any procedure that involves a risk of a health state worse than would be experienced without treatment; because this is often clinically impossible, this strategy often recommends doing nothing unless a sure cure is available.

In Mr. P.'s case, as the worst result under the available choices is early mortality, and early mortality is more likely under watchful waiting (29%) than surgery (10%), a minimax strategy also suggests surgery.

Maximax

If a minimaxer always sees the glass as half empty, the maximaxer always sees it as half full. The maximax strategy is to "maximize the maximum gain" – to choose the option that offers, however unlikely, the best result. For example, given a choice between a procedure that has a 10% chance of death and a 90% chance of cure and another with a 50% chance of partial failure (making their condition somewhat worse) and a 50% chance of partial cure (making their condition somewhat better), the true maximaxer will select the former procedure.

In Mr. P.'s case, the best result under each choice is symptom-free life without early mortality. Accordingly, a maximax strategy suggests watchful waiting, which has the greatest likelihood of resulting in this outcome (67% vs. 66% for surgery).

Minimizing regret

Regret minimizing is a different approach to decision making altogether. A regret minimizer asks himself, "How would I feel if I made this choice and things turned out badly?" Because regret is not simply a reflection of the expected value of the options, but also includes such considerations as how surprising a bad outcome would be, and how responsible the patient would feel for the outcome as a result of their choice, regret-minimizing strategies can result in substantially different decisions.

---

[11] Or the "reasonable worst case." Even minimaxers regularly ignore possibilities that are highly unlikely.

For example, Mr. P. might conclude that it would be much worse to die from cancer knowing that he had not done all he could to treat it than to die from cancer (or experience a poor long-term outcome) after taking the actions available to him to seek a cure (e.g., undergoing surgery or other treatment).

There are good arguments for trying to anticipate regret and similar postdecision emotions. Because it is these feelings that are experienced, perhaps achieving the best feelings is preferable to achieving the highest utility or expected utility. On the other hand, minimizing regret can also be dangerous, particularly when people find bad outcomes due to *action* to be more regrettable than bad outcomes due to *inaction*, a pattern of responses that has been referred to as "omission bias." For example, research has shown that some people would refuse to vaccinate their children if the vaccination itself has a chance of causing death, even when that chance is *lower* than the chance of death from disease for an child left unvaccinated (Ritov and Baron, 1990; Asch *et al.*, 1994).

Using gist

Psychologist Valerie Reyna and her colleagues have argued that more attention should be paid to the representations of outcomes and probabilities in memory rather than their combination at the time of decision. Her research focuses on a model of memory called "fuzzy trace theory" (FTT; Brainerd and Reyna, 1992; Reyna, 2004). The FTT is a dual-process memory model; according to FTT, our memories record both the verbatim details of events and information and a fuzzy or "gist" representation that includes only very rough qualitative features of the information. For example, the gist of Mr. P.'s options might be illustrated by Table 6.4.

As the table shows, each outcome's gist might consist of a rough characterization of the probability and a rough characterization of the value. Very small probabilities are essentially treated as "none," and moderate probabilities may be lumped together as "maybe" or "likely," depending on whether they're more than 50%. Similarly, outcomes are broadly characterized.

Reyna and colleagues argue that in most decisions, the gist representation is activated first and is the primary focus of decision making. Moreover, in many cases, it obviates the need for consideration of difficult trade-offs. For example, on the basis of the representation in Table 6.4, watchful waiting appears the obvious and transparent better choice.

Although the verbatim representation is also present, it is more effortful to retrieve and use and thus less likely to be involved in decision making. Reyna and colleagues not only demonstrate how use of gist results in decisions that systematically differ from maximizing subjective expected value, but also suggest that gist-based decision making is adaptive, and can in fact represent the highest development of reasoning. For example, in a study of medical students, residents, and attending physicians with a wide range of expertise in cardiac care, Reyna and Lloyd (2006) found that the more expert respondents performed best

Table 6.4 Sample long-term outcome gist of radical prostatectomy and watchful waiting

	Probability estimate	Value (0–100)
Radical prostatectomy outcomes		
Complete cure (no significant tumor reappearance or progression before death would occur of other causes)	Likely	Perfect
Cure with permanent erectile dysfunction	Maybe	Fair
Cure with permanent urinary incontinence	Maybe	Fair
Tumor reappearance leading to early mortality	Maybe	Bad
Watchful waiting outcomes		
No significant tumor progression before death would occur of other causes	Likely	Perfect
Tumor progression leading to permanent erectile dysfunction	None	Fair
Tumor progression leading to permanent urinary incontinence	None	Fair
Tumor progression leading to early mortality	Maybe	Bad

at estimating cardiac risk but used less information in their management decisions.

Summary

Two principles are important in decision making with uncertain outcomes. The expectation principle states that a decision maker should attempt to maximize his or her SEU (or other measure of goals) in each decision taken. The preparation principle states that once a decision is taken, the decision maker should consider the range of possible outcomes and prepare for them. In practice, patients make decisions using a variety of strategies, most of which are unlikely to maximize their long-term goals; physicians thus have an opportunity to provide meaningful benefit to patient decision making by examining and improving their decision strategies.

Questions for clinical practice

- What are the expected, or average, outcomes that my patient will receive under each treatment option?
- Once a treatment option is selected, what are the actual outcomes that my patient should prepare for?
- If my patient does not use the expectation principle, how might she or he be making decisions? Could these approaches result in poorer outcomes?

Confidence

Introduction

Mr. R. is seeing his physician because his blood pressure was elevated on a recent life insurance physical. The physician, Dr. M., confirmed his elevated pressure on three different occasions and, based on this information, made the diagnosis of hypertension. On testing, Mr. R. was also found to have an elevated total cholesterol and a low HDL cholesterol level. His doctor asked Mr. R. to come in to the office so that they could discuss treatment of his blood pressure.

Dr. M.: You know Mr. R., the reason I am so interested in working with you to lower your blood pressure is that you can reduce your risk of heart attack and stroke. This seems to me to be a good goal and one I can help you with.

Mr. R.: That sounds like a good goal, doctor, but how high is my risk if I don't do anything for my blood pressure?

Dr. M.: Seeing that you are 55 years old, don't have diabetes, don't smoke, but do have a total cholesterol of 286, which is high, an HDL of 32, which is low, and your blood pressure has been averaging 146/80, I can predict that you have a 19% chance of a either having a heart attack or dying of a heart attack in the next 10 years.[1]

Mr. R.: That is high. I can see your point, but how confident are you in this prediction for me? Is that 19% chance a sure thing or a pretty fuzzy guess? How certain is it that treatment will lower this number?

Determining the best choice to achieve a goal is not always enough to complete a decision. Often, a physician, policy maker, or patient is also concerned with how confident they should be that the recommended choice is superior

---

[1] Calculated using the Risk Assessment Tool at http://hp2010.nhlbihin.net/atpiii/calculator.asp?usertype = prof, based on Antonopoulos (2002).

to other options, and the conditions under which another option would be recommended instead.

The term *confidence* is regularly used in at least two ways in medical decision making: as a statistical statement about uncertainties and as a phenomenological statement about the subjective feeling of accuracy or lack of conflict in a judgment.[2] This chapter discusses both statistical and subjective confidence.

Statistical confidence

"Confidence" has a particular and peculiar meaning in statistics. Researchers typically try to describe the degree of "uncertainty about uncertainty" by providing ranges or bounds on any probability they describe. The most common approach is to give "confidence intervals"; for example, the probability of an allergic reaction to a drug found in a clinical trial may be described as 3% with a 95% confidence interval (95% CI) ranging from 1% to 5%. The meaning of a confidence interval is not entirely intuitive. This 95% CI means that there is a 95% chance that the interval found in the study (1% to 5%) contains the true probability. Of course, there is conversely a 5% chance that the interval does not include the true probability, but scientific convention tends to discount events that occur 5% of the time or less.

Although confidence intervals are valuable in describing the range of an uncertainty, they are confusing to patients and many nonstatisticians, for two reasons. First, the confidence interval itself is described by a percentage (e.g., 95% CI or 99% CI), and this percentage is easily confused with the actual, medical uncertainty of interest. The percentage in the confidence interval (e.g., 95%) is chosen by scientific convention, and has no bearing on the actual uncertainty in the decision.

Second, the 95% CI is easily misinterpreted as meaning that it is 95% likely that the true probability lies between 1% and 5%. This is not the case. The true value either lies in the interval or doesn't; it can't "maybe" lie in the interval. The true value of the probability is fixed – we just do not know this true value. The confidence interval tells us that we have estimated a numerical interval which has a 95% chance of containing the true value. It is our estimate of this true value that is uncertain and around which the confidence interval is formed. In addition, this misinterpretation suggests that the true value of the probability must be at least near that range, which is not the same as the idea that it is 95% likely that the interval 1% to 5% contains the true probability (which may actually be anywhere outside that range).

---

[2] Confidence is also used in a third way, as a synonym for trust, for example, "the patient's confidence in his physician" or "the physician's confidence in her patient's ability to follow directions." This sort of confidence can also be important in implementing medical decisions but is not considered in this chapter.

This misinterpretation of a confidence interval is a natural consequence of difference between frequentist and Bayesian statistics, the two primary approaches to probability and statistics. For frequentists, probability expresses the relative frequency of an event; for Bayesians, probability expresses the subjective belief in an event. A statement that it is 95% likely that the true probability lies between 1% and 5% is a subjective belief referred to as a "credible interval" among Bayesian statisticians. Credible intervals are not regularly computed in biomedical research, both because Bayesian methods are not widely used, and because such methods often require more detailed data than non-Bayesian approaches.[3]

The 95% CI gets particularly confusing if we are talking about the 95% CI for a probability as we are doing in this chapter. When explaining confidence intervals, it often helps to consider the 95% CI around a physical measure, instead, such as the distance of Barry Bonds' record-breaking 756th home run. Imagine that we buy a very long tape measure and fix one end to home plate and stretch the other end to the point of impact of the baseball. We do this same procedure 100 different times and although we are very careful we get different measurements each time (because we're not perfect, because the tape measure expands and contracts with changes in humidity, etc.), From these data we calculate a mean estimated distance. For such physical measurements, which are normally distributed, we can further calculate a standard deviation of our measurements, a standard error of our estimate, and the 95% CI of the mean we have calculated from our 100 measurements. Because it's a 95% CI, we expect that five of our home run measurements will be outside the confidence interval; any (or none) of the 100 measurements could be the true home run ball distance. We cannot say that there is a 95% chance that the true value is inside the interval as the true value of the home run distance is a fixed value and is either inside or outside the interval. We can say that there is a 95% chance that the interval we calculated contains the true measurement.

Confidence intervals are nevertheless quite useful in characterizing the statistical reliability of an estimate. For example, in cost-effectiveness analysis (see Chapter 12), it is common to use a computer to simulate prior distributions of model parameters (costs, outcomes, etc.) and to construct confidence intervals around the probability that one intervention will be more cost-effective than others. They are also regularly used in the research literature to graphically display the precision of an estimate.

For example, Dr. M.'s estimate of Mr. R.'s 10-year risk of a heart attack is 19%. This estimate is based on a well-studied risk factor model applied to a population of patients (Wilson et al., 1998; Lloyd-Jones et al., 2004). For any particular patient, however, the model prediction is only an estimate. If the 95%

---

[3] Specifically, Bayesian statistics often require knowledge of distributions of prior probabilities: *before* the study was conducted, how likely was it that individual patients would have allergic reactions to the drug? These distributions are difficult to estimate in many cases.

CI around the estimate ranges from 15% to 24%, Dr. M. can inform Mr. R. that he is quite certain that this range contains Mr. R.'s actual 10-year risk.

Subjective confidence

Subjective confidence is different from statistical confidence. It is usually thought of as the degree to which a person believes they are correct about a judgment and are willing to say so. Subjective confidence can be important when there is no objective guide to accuracy; in these cases, decision makers usually prefer to make the judgment in which they have the greatest confidence; therefore, subjective confidence can not only drive judgments, it can motivate an individual's further behaviors (Weber *et al.*, 2000). Subjective confidence is also a tool that people often use to check on the accuracy of decisions that are objectively guided. Many decision makers want a decision not only to be logical but to feel right. Accordingly, there has been some concern that decision makers have appropriate levels of confidence in their judgments – because either over- and underconfidence could result in suboptimal decisions.

Subjective confidence can be measured in several ways. People are regularly asked to state their confidence verbally or numerically: "Just how sure are you of that?" Confidence in an outcome is also measured behaviorally, and perhaps more objectively, by asking how willing someone is to take a bet that the outcome they predict will actually occur. A person who is willing to take a bet that pays $10 if they are correct but costs them $50 if they are wrong must be quite confident that they are correct, because they are willing to accept a gamble at 5:1 odds against the outcome.

For example, Dr. M. might tell Mr. R., that although he can never be completely certain, he feels very confident that successful treatment for high blood pressure will reduce Mr. R.'s 10-year risk of heart attack by one third (to 13%). Dr. M. might express this confidence numerically ("Personally, I'm 90% sure that we'll be able to achieve that"). An insurer would be likely to express confidence in this treatment plan by covering it (effectively displaying willingness to gamble up to the cost of the treatment on the effectiveness of the treatment).

Overconfidence and underconfidence

"Overconfidence" is characterized by being more certain of an outcome than appropriate; it is often observed by asking people to give a range of outcomes that they believe has a given (e.g., 95%) chance of including the true outcome and measuring how often their range does, in fact, include the true outcome. That is, people are asked to produce a confidence interval, and overconfidence is measured by examining whether, over a series of these intervals, the true value is included within the interval with the right frequency.

For example, someone might be asked to provide estimates of the number of cars that the five largest automobile manufactures (GM, Toyota, Daimler/Chrysler, Ford, Volkswagen) produced in the first quarter of 2007 along with ranges for each company that they believe has a 95% chance of including the true production. The person who is overconfident in his or her knowledge of car production likely will choose 95% intervals that are too narrow and fail to capture the true value more than the expected 5% of the time. In short, the overconfident decision maker believes he is correct more often than he is.

Overconfidence in medical judgment, particularly in diagnosis, can retard a physician's ability to incorporate new and conflicting information into a diagnostic workup, and can lead to missing important diagnostic cues. Conversely, the underconfident decision maker believes he is correct less often than he is, and provides unnecessarily wide ranges around estimates. Underconfidence in medical decision making can lead to decision paralysis, in which the decision maker never feels that her judgments are sufficiently reliable to take action; when forced to make a choice nonetheless, the decision maker experiences feelings of anxiety and worry.

Calibration

When considering a person's subjective estimate of probability one naturally wonders how accurate that person is. An important measure of the accuracy of someone's confidence judgments is his or her "calibration." Calibration refers to the relationship between the numerical confidence than an event will occur and the actual frequency with which the event occurs.

A meaningful definition of good calibration is one that looks at how well the person judges the likelihood of an event across all situations (Blattenberger and Lad, 1985) and not just in one single and global situation. For example, imagine that we followed a group of 100 patients presenting to the emergency room with chest pain whom the attending physician has admitted to the hospital because he judged that these patients had a 30% chance (each) of myocardial infarction (MI). The next day we determine that 30 of those 100 patients actually had suffered an MI. We might say that the physician is calibrated in his judgments. That is, when he estimates that a patient has a 30% probability of MI, it accurately reflects a 30% chance of MI.

But to really make statements about the calibration of his judgment we need to know more; it is not sufficient to examine only one group or some particular event or events. If the emergency room physician estimated the same 30% MI probability for a 21-year-old man with chest pain after falling off his bicycle as for a 68-year-old man with a long history of diabetes and hypertension who now presents with shortness of breath and crushing chest pain, we would not be impressed at the physician's judgments. Similarly, a physician may be correct when he judges that 10% of adult patients with sore throats have streptococcal pharyngitis, but still show himself to be poorly calibrated when he can't differentiate a high-probability case (a patient with fever, adenopathy, and tonsillar exudates) from a low-probability case (without these findings). We can best assess the physician's calibration when we examine all of the physician's probability judgments, across a large number of patients and situations, and then compare these estimates to the actual frequency of the outcomes.

Being well calibrated is a challenge for physicians and although they can be correct in their global estimate of probability, it is being correct in a specific situation that is important to the patient. An example of being able to make a correct global estimate of probability but still fail to discriminate between high-risk and low-risk cases was reported by Ebell *et al.* (1996). Physicians who are routinely involved in helping patients make advance directives need to be able to give their patients accurate estimates of survival with CPR. Ebell and colleagues asked physicians to read standardized chart abstracts from hospitalized patients who had undergone CPR. Based on these abstracts, these physicians had to estimate the probability of survival following CPR for individual patients. Globally, the physicians were remarkably accurate in estimating the percentage of the patients who survived cardiac arrest with CPR. However, these physicians also assigned similar probabilities of survival to all the patients: those patients who actually survived and those who died. In other words, the physicians could make an accurate global estimate but could not make accurate probability estimates at the patient level.

The examination of calibration is thus challenging because it requires a large number of estimates across a varied population. The result of such a study frequently takes the form of a calibration curve, as illustrated in Figure 7.1. In this figure, the straight diagonal line represents perfect calibration: for any given subjective probability, the observed frequency of the event is identical. The solid line marked with squares illustrates a general underconfidence; the observed frequency is always higher than the subjective probability. In contrast, the dashed line marked with triangles illustrates overconfidence, particularly for more frequently observed events; for example, events with a subjective probability of 99% actually occur only about 75% of the time.

Some researchers distinguish two kinds of overconfidence: "overprediction" and "overextremity" (Griffin and Brenner, 2004). "Overprediction" is a general bias toward giving too high a confidence rating; the overconfident curve shown in Figure 7.1 is an example of overprediction – the subjective probability is always higher than the observed frequency. "Overextremity" is a bias toward giving overly extreme probability values – too high a subjective probability when the observed frequency is high and too low a subjective probability when the observed frequency is low. Similar distinctions can be made between underprediction and underextremity.

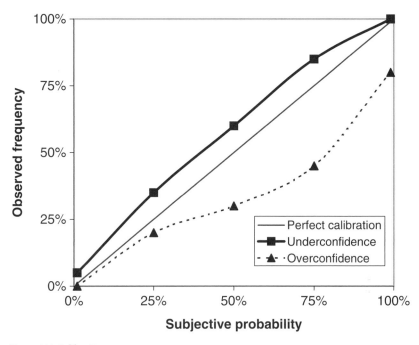

Figure 7.1 Calibration curves.

One group that is regularly called upon to make confidence judgments about uncertain events is weather forecasters, and weather forecasters have been shown to be remarkably well-calibrated in judgments of short-term probability of precipitation and temperature (Murphy and Winkler, 1984; Stewart, Roebber, and Bosart, 1997). Several factors may explain this superior performance. Weather involves fairly well-understood physical processes, and forecasters have access to models of these processes. Weather forecasters make explicit forecasts of common events like precipitation regularly and receive regular and timely feedback on their forecasting success. Finally, weather forecasts are truly exogenous; forecasts do not themselves affect the forecasted events (i.e., the weather). When predicting unusual weather events such as tornado watches, however, weather forecasters are much less well calibrated (Murphy and Winkler 1982; Koehler, Brenner, and Griffin, 2002).

Although calibration of subjective confidence focuses on the physician's expression of confidence in their judgment, it is also possible to examine the calibration of a prediction rule, such as the Framingham risk factor model that Dr. M. applies in his discussion with Mr. R. Studies of the application of that model across many different populations has found that it is quite well-calibrated for patients in the United States, Australia, and New Zealand, but has a tendency toward overprediction for patients in Europe. That is, it predicts a higher risk of cardiac events than are actually found to occur (Eichler *et al.*, 2007).

Improving calibration

Simply informing people about the phenomenon of overconfidence has little effect on their calibration. On the other hand, providing calibration feedback, in which judges are shown their own calibration curves, has been found to be effective in reducing overconfidence and improving calibration (Sieck and Arkes, 2005). Unfortunately, such feedback is difficult to provide in the context of clinical medicine, in which patients are usually encountered and considered individually and physicians frequently do not obtain feedback on their judgments.

More clinically promising approaches include discussion and searching for conflicting evidence. Koriat, Lichtenstein, and Fischhoff (1980) reduced overconfidence by asking people to consider conflicting evidence that would weigh against their initial belief. Arkes, Shaffer, and Medow (1987) showed that group discussion with peers could improve calibration as well. Both of these techniques encourage deeper consideration of choice alternatives and allow for the combination of multiple viewpoints (Weber *et al.*, 2000; Armstrong, 2001); moreover, collegial discussion of cases is a venerable tradition in medicine and occurs naturally in most group practices. What is important in such discussions is to ensure that an effort is made to look for contradictory and disconfirming evidence, not only evidence that confirms or increases confidence in the initial judgment. Sadly, despite promising methods of improving physicians' probability calibration, some studies suggest that simply helping physicians to become better calibrated may not significantly impact their treatment decisions. In one study, physicians taught to make more accurate estimates of the likelihood of a strep throat infection did not reduce their use of antibiotics (Poses *et al.*, 1985; Poses, Cebul, and Wigton, 1995).

Confidence and conflict

Although most people think of confidence as a statement about belief in the accuracy of a judgment, Weber *et al.* (2000) provided a convincing demonstration that confidence may instead reflect a lack of conflict about the decision. In their study, they asked 84 physicians to generate most likely and second most likely diagnoses for cases and to give their confidence in each diagnosis and in the proposition that the correct diagnosis was somewhere in their set. Confidence in the set should always be higher than confidence in any single diagnosis (and it was); moreover, if confidence reflects belief in accuracy of judgment, the confidence in the set should be higher when the top two diagnoses are both likely than when one is likely and the other considerably less likely. Instead, confidence was reduced when the top two diagnoses were both judged to be quite likely.

The authors conclude that expressions of confidence may actually be expressions of a lack of decision conflict. When there is only one likely diagnosis, the confidence in the set is high, because there is little conflict about which diagnosis is correct. When there are two likely diagnoses, however, there is much more conflict about which is *the* most likely diagnosis, and this is reflected in a lower overall confidence for the set. In support of this theory, physicians who mentioned a rival hypothesis when discussing their reasoning for selecting their most likely diagnoses also tended to have lower confidence in that diagnosis (as well as in the set of diagnoses).

Confidence, evidence, and expertise

Although both novices and experts may express confidence, these statements do not have the same import. Experts who are highly confident tend to be right; when not confident, their judgments tend not to be associated with outcomes (McNeil et al., 1982; Friedman et al., 2001). In contrast, confidence judgments of medical students are not related to whether they have correctly or incorrectly diagnosed a case.

However, even expert judgment is sensitive to features of the judgment domain. Research on medical judgments by physicians have found that when making judgments of high-probability events, physicians tend to underpredict the events. When making judgments of low-probability events, physicians tend to be well-calibrated when the events are highly discriminable (there is considerable evidence available to the physician that is relevant to making the judgment) but to overpredict when events are poorly discriminable. This pattern of responses can be explained by assuming that confidence judgments, particularly by experts, represent measures of the amount and quality of supporting evidence for the judgment (Koehler et al., 2002). When the physician can find many arguments in favor of a diagnosis, she will be highly confident in the diagnosis.

Summary

Both patients and physicians are more comfortable about their decisions when they are confident that there are no options superior to the one they have chosen. Moreover, decision makers usually prefer to make the judgment in which they have the greatest confidence. Both statistical and subjective confidence provide useful information about decision recommendations, despite concerns about subjective under- and overprediction. Making the appropriate treatment judgment is linked to good probability calibration, but good calibration is not sufficient.

Questions for clinical practice

- When I provide patients with estimates, such the likelihood that their disease will progress or a treatment will be successful, would they benefit from knowing the statistical confidence interval around the estimate?
- When I provide patients with estimates, how (subjectively) confident am I in my estimate, and why?
- Are there opportunities to improve my confidence judgments (or those of my associates) by getting regular feedback about calibration or creating systems to ensure that disconfirming evidence will be considered?

Part IV

Developing information

Visualizing decisions

Introduction

> Pat and Sam are a married couple with no children. Each is 35 years old, and they are expecting their first child in about 6 months. They are concerned about the possibility of having a child with Down's syndrome. Their obstetrician has offered them the option of having an amniocentesis, having a "quadruple screen" serum test (a blood test measuring serum α-fetoprotein, human chorionic gonadotropin, unconjugated estriol, and inhibin), possibly followed by amniocentesis if the quadruple screen is positive, or skipping testing altogether.

One of the most powerful classes of decision aids are tools for making options, outcomes, and attributes visually comprehensible. This chapter introduces several different kinds of decision visualization and communication tools and develops a vocabulary and taxonomy for creating and evaluating new tools. Particular attention is given to tools for constructing choice sets, weighing and evaluating attributes, and representing the structure of decisions.

Constructing strategies

At first, Pat and Sam seem to have three choices; their obstetrician has informed them that they can have a blood test, an amniocentesis, or no testing. However, these initial decisions can lead to further decisions. A "strategy" refers to a complete sequence of decisions – a full guideline from the initial decision to the final outcome. Pat and Sam have many more than three strategies, some of which are shown in Table 8.1.

In principle, some of the strategies can be excluded as they may be obviously unacceptable to Pat and Sam. For example, strategy 8, terminating the pregnancy without any testing, is clearly an unacceptable strategy, because they desire to have a child. Strategy 4 in the table, in which the pregnancy termination decision is based solely on the quadruple screen, is similarly unlikely to be appropriate; given the relative safety (to the mother) of amniocentesis, risking a small chance

Table 8.1 Selected strategies for Pat and Sam

1. Have no testing and continue the pregnancy
2. Have amniocentesis
   If amniocentesis positive, terminate the pregnancy
   If amniocentesis negative, continue the pregnancy
3. Have amniocentesis
   Regardless of result, continue the pregnancy
4. Have blood test
   If blood test positive, terminate the pregnancy with no further testing
   If blood test negative, continue the pregnancy with no further testing
5. Have blood test
   Regardless of result, continue the pregnancy with no further testing
6. Have blood test.
   If blood test positive, have amniocentesis
   If amniocentesis positive, terminate the pregnancy with no further testing
   If amniocentesis negative, continue the pregnancy with no further testing
   If blood test negative, continue the pregnancy
7. Have blood test.
   If blood test positive, have amniocentesis
   Regardless of result, continue the pregnancy
   If blood test negative, continue the pregnancy with no further testing
8. Terminate pregnancy without any testing

of a procedure-related miscarriage to rule out Down's syndrome seems more reasonable than terminating the pregnancy for certain on the basis of a weaker test.

Although it is a basic principle of decision making that one should not conduct a test if it will not influence a decision, this ignores the value of information itself – people seeking testing not to change what they will do but to mentally prepare for what they will need to do. Strategies 5 and 7, in which the couple will continue the pregnancy regardless of the results of tests, may be sensible in this context. For example, knowing or suspecting that their child may have Down's syndrome may enable Pat and Sam to better prepare psychologically for their role as parents to such a child, or may lead them to seek greater support. Conversely, knowing that their child does not have Down's syndrome may provide greater freedom from worry and anxiety.

One useful way to construct strategies to compare is to draw a picture of the decisions that the patient may face, using arrows to indicate the order in which the decisions can be taken. Figure 8.1 illustrates this process. At the outset, there are two possible choices that can be made: to ship testing, to undergo the quadruple screen, to undergo amniocentesis, or to terminate the

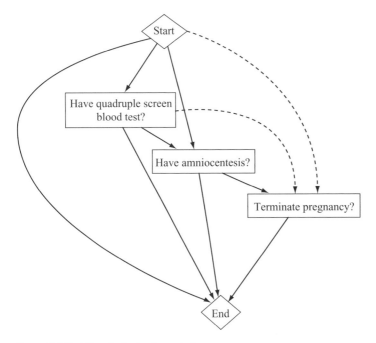

Figure 8.1 Building strategies from choices.

pregnancy. If quadruple screen is chosen, amniocentesis can follow but not vice versa.

Each path from the "start" to "end" in the choice diagram represents a strategy. In the example, there are eight strategies:

1. no testing
2. quadruple screen only (continue the pregnancy regardless)
3. quadruple screen followed (if positive) by termination
4. quadruple screen followed (if positive) by amniocentesis (and then continue the pregnancy regardless)
5. quadruple screen followed (if positive) by amniocentesis followed (if positive) by termination
6. amniocentesis only (and then continue the pregnancy regardless)
7. amniocentesis followed (if positive) by termination
8. unconditional termination

The paths represent all of the strategies listed in Table 8.1. Dashed arrows designate the unrealistic strategies of unconditional termination and termination following positive quadruple screen only and are included for completeness; in practice, unrealistic or unacceptable paths could simply be left out or erased.

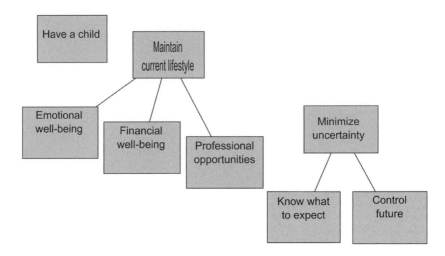

Figure 8.2 A goal map.

Weighing attributes

Having examined their initial set of decisions and the possible strategies they could select, Pat and Sam must also determine their goals in the decision and develop and prioritize the attributes they will use to evaluate their outcomes. Methods for developing goals and attributes were introduced in Chapters 1, 2, and 3; in this chapter, we focus on visualization.

Goals and attributes can be naturally visualized in a hierarchical tree, a method often used in the early stages of the analytic hierarchy process discussed in Chapter 2. For example, Pat and Sam's goals in their decision making might be:

• Have a child.
• Maintain their current lifestyle.
• Minimize uncertainty about the future.

Although having a child is a goal that is either achieved or not, the other goals involve multiple attributes that can each vary in their level of achievement. For example, maintaining one's current lifestyle might include such attributes as financial well-being, emotional well-being, and professional opportunities; all of these will be affected to some degree by pregnancy and childbirth. Similarly, minimizing uncertainty includes both knowing what to expect from the future and controlling what will happen in the future. Figure 8.2 presents a map illustrating the hierarchy of goals and attributes; in this figure, the most important goals appear nearer the top, and less important goals below them.

Pat and Sam may also have constraints; for example, they may not believe in terminating a pregnancy for any reason, or they may not believe in terminating a pregnancy unless the mother's life is endangered. These should also be represented, and assigned importance: are these non-negotiable constraints, or can they be traded off to achieve other goals?

Evaluating attributes of outcomes

Pat and Sam face several possible outcomes, depending on their choice of strategy. These include:
- Bear a healthy child.
- Bear and raise a child with Down's syndrome.
- Bear a child with Down's syndrome who does not survive infancy.
- Miscarry a child with Down's syndrome.
- Terminate a pregnancy to avoid carrying a child with Down's syndrome.

Using their map of goals, Pat and Sam can consider each outcome in turn and use the map either to decompose the outcome into attributes and assign value to it, or to (holistically) consider the outcome in light of their goals and assign it a value. As a result of this process, they might assign a value of 100 to bearing a health child, 80 to raising a child with Down's syndrome, 30 to terminating a pregnancy, 20 to miscarrying a child with Down's syndrome during pregnancy, and 0 to bearing a child with Down's syndrome who dies in infancy.

Visualizing decisions

Pat and Sam now have all the information they need to construct a representation of the decision as a whole that they can use to guide them in choosing a strategy. This representation should bring together all they know about their options. For each option, they know its sequence in each strategy, its possible outcomes, and the probabilities of those outcomes (which might be visualized using the graphical approaches to communicating uncertainty discussed in Chapter 5). For each outcome, they know its utility – how its attributes stack up in terms of achieving their goals.

Pro and con lists

A very familiar and surprisingly useful approach to visualizing decisions is to enumerate, for each choice (or sequence of choices), the pros and cons of making that choice. Naturally, the pros and cons should be based on the decision maker's goals and values, and more important advantages and disadvantages (those having greater impact on higher priority values) should be enumerated first.

This process is typically holistic and noncompensatory (i.e., it does not emphasize trade-offs between values) and will thus sometimes result in choices that do not maximize the subjective expected utility of the decision maker. On

Table 8.2 Pro and con list

Strategy	Pros	Cons
3. Have amniocentesis; regardless of result, continue the pregnancy.	Minimizes uncertainty. Provides preparation if fetus has Down's syndrome.	Potential procedure-related loss (1%)
7. Have blood test. If blood test positive, have amniocentesis and regardless of result, continue the pregnancy If blood test negative, continue the pregnancy.	Reduces uncertainty considerably (small chance of false-negative blood test). Provides preparation if fetus has Down's syndrome.	Potential procedure-related loss from amniocentesis (but only if blood test is positive)
6. Have blood test. If blood test positive, have amniocentesis, and terminate the pregnancy if positive. If blood test negative, continue the pregnancy.	Reduces uncertainty considerably (small chance of false-negative blood test). Reduces chance of lifestyle changes due to having child with Down's syndrome.	Potential procedure-related loss from amniocentesis (only if blood test is positive). Potential termination of pregnancy.

the other hand, pro and con lists are often a fast and easy way to identify strategies that are *dominated* – worse than another strategy no matter what – and these can, and should, be eliminated.[1] Pro and con lists also usually point up the key trade-offs in the decision, and they can be given greater attention.

Table 8.2 presents an example pro and con list for Pat and Sam for three of their possible strategies. Note that strategies 6 and 7 share one advantage (the same reduction of uncertainty) and one disadvantage (potential procedure-related loss from amniocentesis). If Pat and Sam consider termination of pregnancy to be worse than bearing a child with Down's syndrome, strategy 6, which results in termination in some cases, will always be worse than strategy 7, which results in bearing a child with Down's syndrome in those same cases. Accordingly,

---

[1] Failure to eliminate dominated options before making choices can result in an unconscious bias in favor of the option(s) that dominate the dominated option. That is, when some options (but not all) dominate one of the options, the dominating options appear relatively more valuable. This phenomenon is called the "attraction effect" or "asymmetric dominance." For example, physicians have been shown to be more likely to select a one medication over another in the presence of a third medication dominated by the first than in the absence of the third medication (Schwartz and Chapman, 1999).

strategy 6 is dominated by strategy 7 and can be eliminated. Conversely, if they consider bearing a child with Down's syndrome to be worse than terminating a pregnancy, strategy 7 is dominated by strategy 6 and can be eliminated. Either way, the dominating strategy should be compared with strategy 3, which is not dominated by either (as that choice involves a trade-off between less uncertainty about fetal status and greater chances of a procedure-related loss).

A particularly powerful variation of a pro and con list is provided by the Ottawa Personal Decision Guide (O'Connor, Jacobsen, and Stacey, 2006). This downloadable form guides the decision maker through four key steps: clarifying the decision (what is to be decided, why, when, and the decision maker's current inclination), identifying decision-making needs (for support, knowledge, values, and certainty), exploring those needs, and planning the next step based on the needs. The "Explore your needs" section includes a pro/con list in which each advantage or disadvantage listed is also assigned an importance value (from zero to five stars), and the choice with the most likely advantages is circled.

Decision trees

Decision trees are the most common tool that decision scientists use to represent the structure of a decision. A decision tree is a way of representing choices, uncertainties, and potential outcomes. Figure 8.3 depicts a simplified decision tree for a hypothetical medical decision: should a patient presenting symptoms of some disease receive drug treatment or undergo surgery? Assume that if treatment is not successful, the patient will die. Drug treatment has only a 50% chance of success but, if successful, will restore the patient to full health. Surgery has a 75% chance of saving the patient, but as a result of the surgery, the patient will be left with some limitations on his or her future activities.

Square nodes represent decisions, circular nodes represent uncertainties, and triangular nodes represent outcomes. Time in decision trees flows from left to right. First, a decision will be made between drug treatment and surgery. If drug treatment is chosen, there is an uncertainty: will treatment be successful

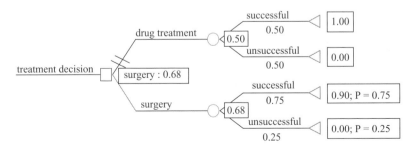

Figure 8.3 A simplified treatment decision tree.

or unsuccessful? The probabilities of each possibility are drawn underneath its branch; in this case, there is a 0.50 probability of success. If the drug treatment is successful, the patient will receive an outcome with value 1.00, representing full heath. If the treatment fails, the patient will die, which is conventionally assigned the value 0.

Similarly, if surgery is elected, it may be successful (with a 0.75 probability) or unsuccessful (0.25 probability). If successful, the results have value 0.90; the patient is not fully restored to health but is still quite well off. If unsuccessful, the patient dies.

If the decision maker's goal is to maximize expected utility, the decision tree can be "solved" to yield an optimal set of decisions. Decision trees are solved by a process of working backward, applying simple expected value calculations. The expected value of drug treatment is the probability of success (0.50) multiplied by the value of success (1.00), plus the probability of failure (.50) multiplied by the value of failure (0), which totals 0.50. The expected value of surgery is the probability of success (0.75) multiplied by the value of success (0.90), plus the probability of failure (0.25) multiplied by the value of failure (0.00), which totals 0.68. Because the expected value of surgery is higher than the expected value of drug treatment, surgery should be recommended to patients with this disease. This is shown in the tree by crossing out the path that leads to the lower expected value, and writing the higher expected value and the option that yields it in the box next to the decision node.

The probabilities shown by the outcomes of the surgery option on the right side of the tree indicate what proportion of people can be expected to obtain those outcomes if the decision is implemented for a group. In this case, if everyone in the group undergoes surgical treatment, we expect that 75% of them will obtain a health state with value 0.90 and 25% will die.

Computer software exists to automate the process of drawing and solving decision trees. Even without the data required to solve a tree, however, simply sketching out a sequence of decisions and uncertainties in tree form is often very helpful in visualizing a set of decisions that a patient face.

For example, Figure 8.4 illustrates part of the decision facing Pat and Sam. They face a choice between three testing options (no testing, quad screen followed by amniocentesis if positive, and amniocentesis). If they receive a positive amniocentesis result, they face a later decision about whether to terminate the pregnancy. As they move through the tree, their decisions and the resolution of the uncertainties eventually result in one of the outcomes on the right of the tree.

This tree differs from the previous simple tree in that symbolic names like "pDowns" and "uTerminated" are used to represent the probabilities and utilities involved in the decision. The box at the far left of the tree shows the values assigned to each of the symbolic names. Using names rather than numbers is helpful to both patients and decision analysts. Patients can more easily

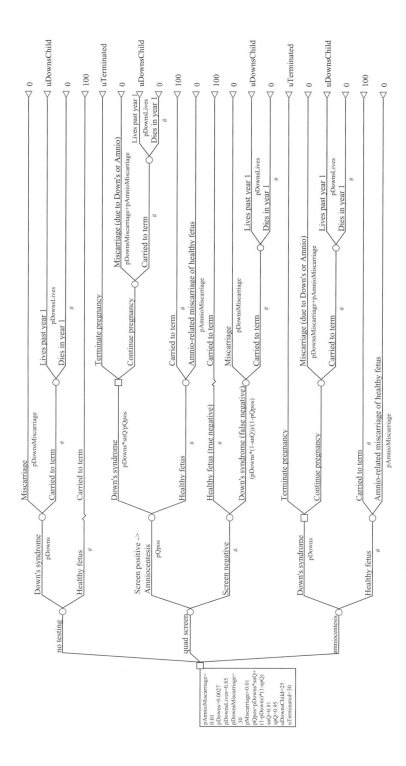

Figure 8.4 Decision tree for prenatal Down's syndrome testing.

distinguish the uncertainties and outcome values when they are named; when only numbers are provided in the tree, it can be laborious to recall the meaning of each number and it's easier to confuse utilities and probabilities. Decision analysts prefer to use symbolic names because they make it simpler to change the model parameters in light of new information. If the probability of miscarriage owing to amniocentesis decreases (e.g., due to improved techniques), the analyst need only change the value of "pAmnioMiscarriage" at the start of the tree rather than search for every instance of "0.01," ensuring that it really is meant to refer to that probability and changing it in the tree.

Influence diagrams

An influence diagram is another way of representing choices, uncertainties, and potential outcomes (Nease 1997; Owens, Shachter, and Nease, 1997). Figure 8.5 depicts a simplified influence diagram for the hypothetical medical decision introduced in the discussion of decision trees.

In an influence diagram, square nodes represent decisions, circular nodes represent uncertainties, and diamond nodes represent outcomes. Arrows drawn from nodes to the outcome assert that the outcome depends on the decisions and uncertainties pointing to it. Arrows drawn from nodes to decisions assert that the information or choice taken in those nodes is known at the time the decision is made. Arrows drawn from nodes to uncertainties assert that the probability associated with the uncertainty depends on the decisions and uncertainties pointing to it. The lack of an arrow between two nodes asserts that the two are independent. In Figure 8.5, the outcome is influenced by the treatment chosen and its success. The success of the treatment depends on the treatment chosen.

The table under the "Success of treatment" node shows the how it depends on the choice of treatment. If drug treatment is chosen, there is a 0.50 probability of success. Similarly, if surgery is elected, it may be successful (with a 0.75 probability) or unsuccessful (0.25 probability).

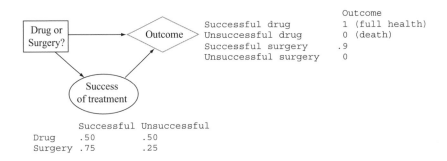

Figure 8.5 A simplified influence diagram.

The table next to the "Outcome" node shows how the outcomes depend on the choice of treatment and success of the treatment. If the drug treatment is successful, the patient will receive an outcome with value 1.00, representing full heath. If the treatment fails, the patient will die, which is conventionally assigned the value 0.00. If surgery is successful, the results have value 0.90; the patient is not fully restored to health but is still quite well off. If unsuccessful, the patient dies.

Influence diagrams are often used by decision analysts to capture information about the relationships between variables and choices in a decision problem. As with decision trees, computer software exists to automate the process of drawing and solving influence diagrams. And, like decision trees, even without the data required to solve an influence diagram, the diagram itself can be a useful way to get a handle on the key decisions and uncertainties that will contribute to the patient's outcome.

The influence diagram for Pat and Sam's prenatal testing decision, shown in Figure 8.6, is considerably more complex, although it still presents key information about the relationships between decisions and uncertainties in a more compact way than a decision tree. In this diagram, the outcome depends on five factors: whether the pregnancy is terminated, whether the fetus is miscarried due to amniocentesis, whether the fetus is miscarried spontaneously, whether the fetus has Down's syndrome, and whether the child dies before 1 year old.

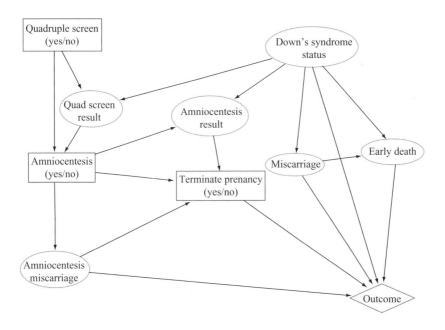

Figure 8.6 Influence diagram for prenatal Down's syndrome testing.

The three decisions – to perform the quad screen, to perform an amniocentesis, and to terminate the pregnancy – are presented with arrows indicating the order in which they occur (quad screen, if chosen, before amniocentesis, and both before termination decisions). There is an arrow from the amniocentesis result to the termination decision but not from the quad screen result, because termination will be based only on the results of amniocentesis.

The influence diagram and decision tree can both be used to visually lay out a decision, although they make different kinds of information salient. The influence diagram shows the connections between the variables more clearly than the decision tree. The decision tree shows details about the paths individuals can take as the decision unfolds, but the decision trees both simplify decisions and increase visual complexity: decision trees typically treat variables as discrete – collapsing them into a small number of alternatives – when they may actually be continuous, and the number of nodes in a decision tree increases exponentially with the number of decision and chance variables. Comparing Figure 8.4 and Figure 8.6 makes this more obvious. The influence diagram provides a much more compact representation of the decision and emphasizes the interconnections in the decision. Although it takes some practice to read an influence diagram, it provides a concise and powerful visual summary of the components of the decision.

Summary

Patients facing significant medical decisions often have difficulty keeping track of all of the associated choices, strategies, uncertainties, and outcomes. Physicians can help patients to visualize their decisions by introducing tools that simplify or clarify the processes of building strategies, weight and evaluating attributes, and comprehending decisions as a whole.

Questions for clinical practice

- Have my patients considered the sequences of choices they may face and constructed a list or map of strategies?
- How can I help my patients to consider the advantages and disadvantages of each of their potential strategies?
- Would a decision tree or influence diagram help my patients to better understand the clinical features of the decisions they face?

The power of information

Introduction

Chris and Robin are a married couple in nearly the same position as Pat and Sam (from Chapter 8), but a few years older. They've tentatively decided to proceed directly with amniocentesis and to terminate the pregnancy if the fetus has Down's syndrome; their alternative was to forgo testing entirely. Before they have the amniocentesis, however, they wonder if there's any better information about the probability of amniocentesis-related miscarriage of a healthy fetus, and how sure they are about their preferences for bearing a child with Down's syndrome versus terminating such a pregnancy.

One of the available options in many decisions is to gather more information. Indeed, it has been argued that in every clinical decision, the set of options to be considered should include, at minimum, wait and see, treat immediately, and collect more information (Hunink, 2005).

We can conceptualize the usefulness of additional information by considering how much a decision recommendation would change (or could be improved) if additional information were available. However, additional information often comes at a cost. This chapter provides both a conceptual and simplified mathematical introduction to the use of information in decisions and offer the clinician strategies for determining which information should be obtained in a decision and when. The chapter also discusses evidence-based medicine (EBM) and the development of clinical trials.

A model decision

We use the case of Chris and Robin as a model decision in which gaining additional information might be valuable. In doing so, we make the following initial assumptions about their clinical situation and preferences:
- The probability that their fetus has Down's syndrome is 2%.
- The probability of procedure-related fetal loss from amniocentesis is 1%.

- Their preference value for bearing a healthy child is 100.
- Their preference value for carrying a fetus with Down's syndrome is 15.
- Their preference value for terminating a pregnancy (when the fetus has Down's syndrome) is 70.[1]

Their decision could be represented by the decision tree shown in Figure 9.1. This tree assumes that amniocentesis results will be known whether or not there is a procedure-related loss and, for simplicity, that the couple's value for a procedure-related loss of a fetus with Down's syndrome is the same as their value for terminating a pregnancy in which the fetus is known to have Down's syndrome.

Based on these assumptions, the expected value for the amniocentesis choice is 98.4; the expected value for the no testing choice is 98.3. Accordingly, amniocentesis should be (slightly) preferred. Because the choice is close, however, Chris and Robin are interested in finding out if there's any further information they could obtain that would clarify the decision.

The second opinion

The most venerable approach to gathering additional information is to consult another physician, often one with expertise in the decision, and obtain a second opinion. For example, if Chris and Robin are particularly concerned with the probability of procedure-related loss from amniocentesis, they might consult another obstetrician who might provide a different estimate.

Differences in opinion may arise from a number of underlying factors. The new consultant may have greater expertise and experience, which may enable her either to provide a more precise or more confident estimate around the risks of existing options or to actually recommend alternative options that might have lower risks. For example, if the consulting obstetrician was aware of a safer technique for sampling fetal chromosomes unknown to their primary obstetrician, she might be able to recommend the new technique as an option.

Differences in opinion may also arise from idiosyncratic differences in physician values, individual differences in risk attitudes and risk perceptions, habitual or regional variations in approach, differential availability of options, and others. These sources of differences in opinion are usually less welcome than differences arising from greater expertise; when two physicians each suspect the other's opinion is based on such external features, the irreconcilable opinions may drive the patient to seeking a third "tie-breaker" opinion. Another option is for Chris and Robin to seek out high-quality information on the Internet from sites such as MedlinePlus or PubMed.

---

[1] For simplicity, these values are assumed to reflect the expected impact that they will experience from having a fetus with Down's syndrome, including such outcomes as spontaneous miscarriage, infant mortality, and lifestyle impact of raising the child should it live past infancy.

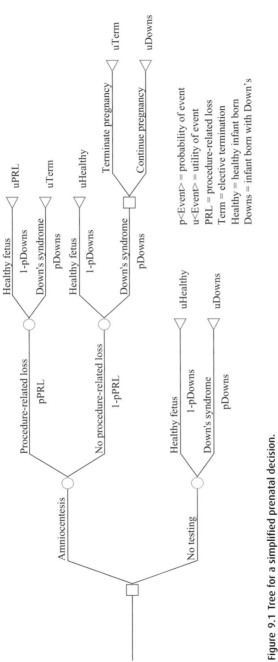

Figure 9.1 Tree for a simplified prenatal decision.

On the other hand, when a second (or third) opinion confirms the original opinion, it can powerfully strengthen the degree of confidence in the diagnosis or recommendation. Psychological research suggests that many kinds of judgments can be made more accurate by aggregating the judgments of multiple experts, or even taking a "majority vote" among experts (as in the case where a "tie-breaker" third opinion is solicited; Yaniv, 2004).

Sensitivity analysis

Sensitivity analysis (not to be confused with the sensitivity of a diagnostic test) is a formal method for examining the impact of changing assumptions on a decision model's recommendation. In effect, a sensitivity analysis involves repeating the decision analysis across a range of assumptions and looking to see if the decision would change.

Chris and Robin have reason to believe that their decision might be sensitive to the probability of procedure-related loss from amniocentesis; if that risk is high enough, they sense that they probably should not undergo amniocentesis. Similarly, if they have experiences that might cause them to reflect on their preferences and revise their preference for carrying a fetus with Down's syndrome upward, they ought to be less likely to favor amniocentesis. Sensitivity analysis can tell them just how much the probability or preference would have to change to make forgoing testing a better option.

Threshold sensitivity analysis

The simplest form of sensitivity analysis is threshold sensitivity analysis. This approach simply examines a range of values for each of the important uncertainties in the model and determines the best choice at each value in the range. For example, Figure 9.2 shows the impact of varying the probability of procedure-related loss from 0.5% to 2%. The diagonally sloping line shows the expected value associated with amniocentesis; the dashed flat line shows the expected value associated with no testing. As the probability of procedure-related loss increases, the value of amniocentesis decreases, and drops below the value of no testing when the probability is 1.1% or higher (the "threshold"). If the average procedure-related loss in national surveys is 1% but the rate varies depending on facility, Chris and Robin might be justifiably concerned with the facility that performs their amniocentesis.

Threshold sensitivity analysis can also be performed for more than one uncertain parameter at once. Analysis on two parameters is easy to visualize; beyond two parameters, visualization becomes more difficult. Figure 9.3 shows the impact of varying both the probability of procedure-related loss and the utility

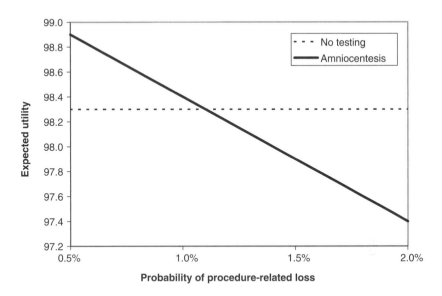

Figure 9.2 Sensitivity analysis of decision tree on one parameter.

of carrying a fetus with Down's syndrome. The parameters appear on the axes, and each combination of the two parameters is a point in the graph. Points in the diagonally cross-hatched region on the left are those where the combination of parameters favors amniocentesis; points in the region on the right are those where the parameters favor no testing.

As the figure illustrates, amniocentesis is favored at lower levels of risk, and at lower levels of preference for carrying a fetus with Down's syndrome. If Chris and Robin's value for carrying a fetus with Down's increases from 15 to a value higher than 21, amniocentesis at its expected 1% rate of procedure-related loss is no longer preferred.

Probabilistic sensitivity analysis

Threshold sensitivity analysis examines the independent and joint impact of changes in parameters on the decision recommendation, but provides no information about how likely different parameter values might be. For example, if the probability of procedure-related loss might lie between 0.5% and 2%, how are those values distributed? Are they all equally likely? Is 1% the most likely value, and then values higher or lower than 1% become increasingly less likely?

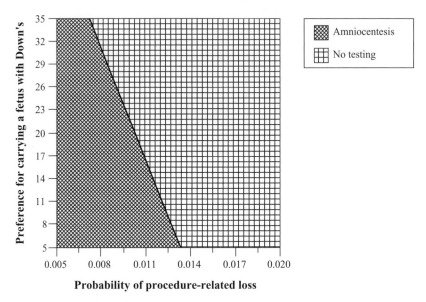

Figure 9.3 Sensitivity analysis of decision tree on two parameters.

Without this kind of information on parameter distributions, a decision may appear to be sensitive to some combination of parameters when in fact that combination is extraordinarily unlikely to occur.

Accordingly, many decision analysts performing sensitivity analysis, particularly for policy-making purposes, use probabilistic sensitivity analysis rather than threshold sensitivity analysis. In a probabilistic sensitivity analysis, the analyst must specify the probability distribution of each parameter or must develop such probability distributions by performing simulations of possible parameter values[2] (Felli and Hazen, 1998).

Figure 9.4 plots three different probability distributions for a single variable. In the uniform distribution (solid horizontal line), the probability varies from 20% to 80% with each value equally likely. In the normal distribution (dotted bell-shaped curve), 50% is the most likely probability, and as probabilities diverge from 50%, they become increasingly less likely. In the exponential

---

[2] Such simulations are typically referred to in the literature as Monte Carlo methods. For example, given probability distributions for three parameters, it would be difficult to develop a joint probability distribution across all the parameters mathematically, but it is simple to have a computer repeatedly generate values of the parameters (each based on its respective probability distribution) and then estimate the ("empirical") joint distribution from these repeated samples.

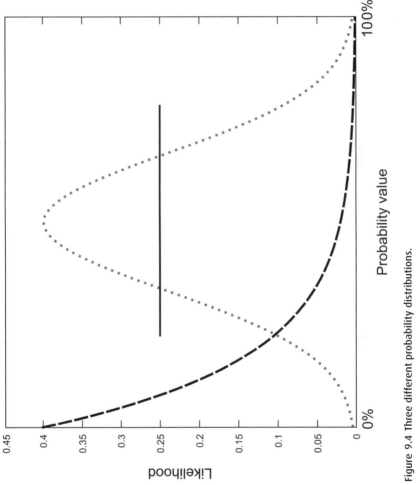

Figure 9.4 Three different probability distributions.

distribution (dashed decreasing curve), small probabilities are much more likely than larger probabilities.

When there is not enough information available to produce a complete (continuous) probability distribution, a rough estimate can be made by constructing a discrete probability distribution – a simple table of the likelihood that the parameter takes on a set of single values. For example, Table 9.1 gives a sample discrete probability distribution for the "rate of procedure-related loss" parameter in Chris and Robin's fetal testing decision. Although a 1% miscarriage rate is the most likely correct estimate, other estimated rates are also assigned a likelihood for the purposes of probabilistic sensitivity analysis.

Although probabilistic sensitivity analysis has major advantages over threshold methods for important decisions, it has two primary disadvantages that make it largely unsuitable for use in a clinical encounter with an individual patient. First, the computations required to perform such analyses, although well within the capability of modern personal computers, are nevertheless time consuming and exacting; probabilistic sensitivity analyses generally cannot be performed by non-experts. More important, it is unclear how one would guide a patient to develop the probability distribution around his or her preferences in the decision. Probabilistic methods are thus likely to be useful in the development of guidelines that can be applied to groups of patients, but threshold methods may be more informative to the individual decision maker.

Value of information analysis

Sensitivity analysis (in both its threshold and probabilistic forms) deals only with the likelihood that parameter changes will result in changes in the decision recommendation. They don't consider either the cost of improving information about a parameter or the impact of the changes on the utility difference between the decision options. That is, a decision could appear to be sensitive to a parameter, but it could make no practical difference, because the cost of gathering more precise information on the parameter is greater than the benefit from improving the decision.

Value of information analysis directly addresses these concerns by asking the question "how much benefit could be expected from improving information on a parameter?" Parameters that will yield a large benefit (the value of information) from additional information at a relatively low cost for acquiring the information are parameters that should be given extra attention by the decision maker. Value of information approaches come in several flavors.

The expected value of information

The expected value of information (EVI) refers to the expected difference between the utility of the best decision possible in light of additional information

Table 9.1 A discrete probability distribution

Presumed rate of procedure-related loss (%)	Likelihood that presumed rate is actual rate (%)
0.5	30
1.0	50
1.5	10
2.0	10

and the utility of the best decision possible without additional information. Computing EVI requires not only probability distributions of the parameters before information gathering but also revised distributions that are expected after information gathering (Meltzer, 2001). As a result, EVI is unlikely to be practically useful in clinical encounters.

The expected value of perfect information

The expected value of perfect information (EVPI) refers to the expected difference between the utility of the best decision under clairvoyance – perfect knowledge about the true values of all the parameters (Howard, 1966) – and utility of the best decision without additional information. Computing EVPI requires probability distributions of parameters before information gathering, but not revised distributions, and is thus more feasible than EVI, but still potentially quite difficult. Because perfect information is an ideal, the EVPI represents an upper bound on the EVI.

More tractable is the so-called partial EVPI (also written EVPXI), which gives the expected value of clairvoyance for a subset of the parameters in the decision (Yokota and Thompson, 2004). For example, it might be practical to ask what the impact of perfect information about the rate of procedure-related loss for amniocentesis would be on Chris and Robin's decision. Given the probability distribution on that parameter, we can ask, for each parameter value, how the expected utility of amniocentesis would change if we knew that was the true rate of loss and determine the expected utility of amniocentesis over the distribution as a whole. Comparing that with the expected utility associated with the best possible decision without that information would yield the expected additional utility that could be obtained from perfect information around that rate.

A simplified (but possibly clinical useful) approach might proceed using the discrete probability distribution from Table 9.1. In Table 9.2, information about utilities has been added to enable the calculation of partial EVPI for the rate of procedure-related loss.

Table 9.2 Approximation of expected value of perfect information

Presumed rate of procedure-related loss (%)	Likelihood that presumed rate is actual rate (%)	Expected utility for amniocentesis under presumed rate (Figure 9.2)	Expected utility for no testing	Difference in expected utilities between best and worst choice	Difference in expected utilities × likelihood
0.5	30	98.9	98.3	0.6	0.18
1.0	50	98.4	98.3	0.1	0.05
1.5	10	97.9	98.3	0.4	0.04
2.0	10	97.4	98.3	**0.9**	0.09
EVPI on rate of procedure-related loss					0.36

The analysis suggests that having perfect information about the rate of procedure-related loss yields, on average 0.36 additional utility points on a 100-point scale (although the actual difference in utility may range from 0.1 to 0.9). This seems a relatively small expected change in potential utility, and a single couple is unlikely to have the means to gather perfect information on this parameter at a cost that would justify the change in utility.[3]

The expected value of imperfect information

Although it is rarely feasible to achieve clairvoyance about a decision parameter, imperfect information is often available. For example, the rate of procedure-related loss might be (imperfectly) predictable by means of a set of risk factors (such as the experience of the obstetrician performing the amniocentesis and the gestational age of the fetus). An analyst can then compute the expected value of imperfect information (EVII): the value associated with gathering these risk factors and using them to provide an improved prediction of the parameter and compare it to the cost of gathering the risk factors (minimal, in this example).[4] Naturally, the EVII cannot exceed the EVPI, but it may be much less costly to obtain.

---

[3] On the other hand, if many couples face this decision, their total utility gain could conceivably be large enough to warrant an investigation to provide better information about this parameter, as the cost of such an investigation is fixed, while the benefit increases with the number of couples who face the decision.

[4] A nonclinical variation of this approach involves choosing the number of patients to include in research study to provide more precise (but still imperfect) values for a parameter. In this variation, it is the expected value of sample information that is computed for the given sample.

The maximum value of information

Computations of EVPI and EVII still require an estimate of the parameter distribution, such as that in Table 9.2. With only a range of values, and no complete probability distribution, EVPI cannot be computed, but the *maximum value of information* (MVI) can be determined. The MVI represents the largest (rather than the expected) difference in utility that could arise if additional information were available on one or more parameters (Meltzer, 2001). For example, examining the range of differences in expected utilities between best and worst choices for procedure-related loss in the fifth column of Table 9.2 reveals that the MVI is 0.9; this results when additional information reveals that the actual rate of loss is 2%, and, as a result, the couple chooses to forgo testing. The MVI is a maximum in that no additional information about procedure-related loss can yield more than 0.9 utility points.

Just as EVPI represents an upper bound on EVI, MVI represents an upper bound on EVPI. Accordingly, it is only really useful when the MVI is small (or small relative to the cost of gathering information), as it then suggests that gathering more information will not be useful for the decision maker. For example, if a difference of 0.9 is small for this decision, gaining additional information on the rate of procedure-related loss will not be helpful, because it cannot result in a meaningful difference in the expected utility to the decision maker.

Table 9.3 summarizes the approaches to deciding when to collect additional information about a clinical problem. Approaches are listed in order from those requiring the most data to compute (which are therefore least likely to be clinical useful) to those requiring the least data to compute.

Clinical research

The primary source of new medical knowledge is medical research. Most clinical research is explicitly motivated by a need to reduce the uncertainties around etiology, prevention, diagnosis, treatment, or prognosis. Principles have been developed to guide the proper design and conduct of clinical research (Brody, 2004).

Although research can extend our knowledge, the effective use of research for reducing clinical uncertainty is not always straightforward. For example, research conducted on the development of new drugs often results in adding a new treatment to the set of available choices that is not universally or unequivocally better than existing treatments. Consequently, this kind of research may actually *increase* uncertainty about the most appropriate treatment for a particular patient, while simultaneously decreasing uncertainty about the availability of *a* suitable treatment.

It has been argued that the development of clinical research itself ought to be an exercise in value-of-information analysis (Claxton, Sculpher, and

Table 9.3 Approaches to deciding when to collect additional information, in order of stringency of required data

Analysis	Data requirements	Provides
Expected value of information (EVI)	Prior and post-information probability distributions for all parameters	Best estimate of utility impact of collecting all possible information
Expected value of perfect information (EVPI)	Prior probability distributions for all parameters	Utility impact of having clairvoyance about all parameters
Partial expected value of perfect information (EVPXI)	Prior probability distributions for one or more parameters of interest	Utility impact of having clairvoyance about one or more parameters
Probabilistic sensitivity analysis	Probability distributions for one or more parameters of interest	Likelihood that recommended option is better than other options
Expected value of imperfect information (EVII)	(Imperfect) means of predicting values of one or more parameters of interest	Utility impact of gathering predictors about one or more parameters
Maximum value of information (MVI)	Range of parameter values for one or more parameters of interest	Maximum possible utility benefit from gaining information on one or more parameters
Threshold sensitivity analysis	Range of parameter values for one or more parameters of interest	Parameter values under which recommended option is better than other options
Second opinion	Same data as available to decision maker, and anything additional requested by second physician	Confirmation that decision is properly structured, and data were properly collected and interpreted; can provide alternative options not yet considered
Subjective confidence in decision (Chapter 7)	None, but more accurate if disconfirming evidence is sought	Personal belief in decision correctness

Drummond, 2002; Claxton, Cohen, and Neumann, 2005). Health research priorities can be set on the basis of which areas of research have the highest EVPI across the proportion of people in society who will benefit from the development of new treatments, tests, or other tools.

This approach has been recently adopted in the United Kingdom by the National Institute for Health and Clinical Excellence (NICE; Claxton and

Sculpher, 2006). For example, recent NICE guidance on the use of cardiac resynchronization included value-of-information analyses to determine what kind of additional utility or cost-utility on a per-patient and population basis could be obtained for a given budget expenditure on research in this area (Fox *et al.*, 2007). The authors conduct one-way threshold sensitivity analyses on many parameters in the cost-effectiveness of CRT-P devices as compared to optimal pharmaceutical therapy (OPT). They find that the cost-effectiveness is particularly sensitive to nine parameters. They also conduct a probabilistic sensitivity analysis that finds that CRT-P will be more cost-effective than OPT under about 95% of the possible combinations of parameter values. Finally, they report that the EVPI to the population for this decision would be 6.2 million British pounds; they argue that this large potential expected value justifies further research in the area.

Even when high-quality research has been performed, identified, and even codified in practice guidelines by professional societies, the results may not be widely adopted by the medical community. There are three primary obstacles to the adoption of new approaches that promise to reduce clinical uncertainty: lack of effective dissemination to practicing physicians, lack of comfort learning an unfamiliar regimen among physicians, and health care system impediments such as cost of care.

At the same time that adoption of proven improvements in medical care is slowed by these difficulties, it has become easier and easier for Internet-savvy patients to obtain information about conditions and treatments – from both trustworthy and untrustworthy sources. Indeed, both the decreased time available for appointments under many health plans and the increased emphasis on patient autonomy in medical decision making exert pressure for patients to "do their homework," often with limited guidance as to how to evaluate the information they develop.

Direct marketing of pharmaceuticals to patients has had a major impact on demand for new drugs in the few countries where it is permitted (Hollon, 1999; Mintzes *et al.*, 2002). Although pharmaceutical advertising is regulated in many countries, and physicians are familiar with marketing strategies used by drug companies, patients may not be as prepared to evaluate advertising claims for pharmaceutical products, much less for the larger group of unregulated supplements and alternative medicine products. Patients who are less well-educated may be at particular risk and face a double jeopardy: they may be less likely to have access to optimal care and less likely to be able to discriminate between safe and risky treatments. Indeed, these concerns have prompted calls for the prohibition of direct-to-consumer pharmaceutical ads in the United States (Stange, 2007).

The combination of slow dissemination of rigorously evaluated medical advances among physicians and rapid dissemination of unscientific advice and claims among patients is a recipe for disaster. Public policy initiatives to improve health literacy among patients are an important strategy to avert catastrophe, but cannot substitute for the impact of effective communication between well-informed physicians and their patients. Physicians can help their patients by taking the lead in explaining how medical research is conducted, suggesting sources of credible information that patients can use, and addressing the strengths and weaknesses of information from whatever source. Patients can help their physicians by learning how to seek out reliable information and bringing it to the clinical encounter with a critical eye.

Evidence-based medicine

No clinician can see every combination of outcomes of the myriad of decisions faced by their patients. Even with substantial experience in a subspecialty, physicians are likely to get only a good sample of possibilities, and, as discussed in Chapter 5, may not be able to accurately recall frequencies of events (much less probability distributions or confidence intervals around such frequencies). Accordingly, as part of their professional responsibilities, clinicians have always sought to keep up with the latest clinical research in their field. Clinical research allows a physician to take advantage of much larger samples of patients and their experiences.

The translation of clinical research to clinical practice faces several obstacles. First, the amount of new clinical research published each year is astounding and shows no sign of decreasing. As a result, merely keeping up with one's field has become a more and more difficult process for physicians, particularly those who do not have ready access to academic medical libraries or online article databases.

In addition, not all research is equal. Many studies are beset with serious, and sometimes fatal, flaws in methods or measurement or greatly overgeneralize their conclusions. Conflict of interest among study researchers is not uncommon.

EBM, an approach advocated in academic medicine since the 1980s, seeks to address these concerns by providing tools and training to permit physicians to focus their limited reading time on research that is methodologically strong and thus likely to yield reliable insights. EBM is an approach to clinical practice that emphasizes using the clinical literature on a "just-in-time" basis to find answers to questions as they arise in clinical practice (Straus *et al.*, 2005).

The practice of EBM involves formulating a well-structured clinical question focused on such matters as the diagnostic value of a particular test or the expected outcomes of alternative treatments for well-defined conditions (e.g., "In a 39-year old pregnant woman at 14 weeks gestation, what is the probability of miscarriage associated with amniocentesis vs. no testing?"). Answers to these questions are sought by searching the medical literature, and search filters may be used to ensure that studies identified are of high methodological quality (Haynes and Wilczynski, 2004; Haynes *et al.*, 2005). Individual studies are rigorously evaluated using standardized criteria to determine how well the study responds to the clinical question that prompted the inquiry.

EBM requires that clinicians learn new skills, including methods for formulating questions about their patients that can be answered in the medical literature, how to search the clinical research literature for potentially relevant research reports, and how to critically appraise the research design and analysis methods to determine the validity of reported results and their applicability to their patients. These skills are not trivial and studies have raised doubts as to how well physicians can master all these tasks. Evidence-based practice also requires an investment in time. Even using current electronic systems, finding and selecting literature-based data to solve a single patient-related problem can easily require an hour or more (Florance, 1996).

On the other hand, once the skills of EBM are mastered, they can be used effectively to focus a physician's reading time on those studies that are most likely to benefit his or her patients, either individually or collectively. The value of the information available from the clinical literature may easily exceed its cost in time when it can be applied to multiple patients.[5]

Summary

Seeking additional information is a common option in medical decisions, particularly consequential decisions that may only be faced once by a given patient. Several techniques have been developed to determine what additional information will have the most impact on the decision, including sensitivity analysis and value of information analysis. Although many of these techniques are highly mathematical to implement fully, some can be approximated in clinically useful ways. More importantly, these methods draw attention to the distinction between the availability of information and its usefulness in decision making. For physicians – who will see many patients – and for the health care system – which seeks to serve them – variations of these approaches can help to guide the use and development of the clinical research knowledge base.

Questions for clinical practice

- What uncertainties could change the decision if more information were available about them?
- What opportunities exist for gathering additional information? Is the cost of doing so worth the potential benefit?
- What sources of information are available from the clinical research literature?

---

[5] Obviously, EBM is limited in its ability to provide information about individual patients and their goals, values, and preferences. It is at its best as a source of data about medical probabilities and outcomes; it cannot be a substitute for one-on-one decision making.

Screening and testing

Introduction

Jane is a 15-year-old high school freshman who has been in good health who came to you for a pre-participation athletic evaluation. She takes no medications, has never been hospitalized, and has had regular menstrual periods since age 13.

She does very well academically and is planning to go out for the cross-country team this year. Eventually, she hopes to be admitted to a highly competitive college on graduation from high school.

Her physical examination was normal, but on routine laboratory testing you found that she had a low hematocrit (35%) and low MCV (74). You asked her to take an iron supplement, which she consistently took twice a day. A month later, her hematocrit and MCV were unchanged and you obtained a serum ferritin level, which was low (18 mg/mL). Further screenings for fecal occult blood and celiac disease were negative.

Because of the unexplained iron-deficiency anemia, you decide to test her for *Helicobacter pylori* infection and consider the use of the noninvasive ^{13}C-urea breath test (UBT) rather than endoscopy. Jane's parents also like the idea of a noninvasive test but want to know how accurate the test is and whether a follow-up endoscopy will be necessary anyway if the breath test is negative.

In many clinical decisions, the most ready source of additional information is diagnostic testing. Diagnostic tests include not only laboratory tests, but other sources of information about diagnosis, such as history and physical examination. We have already seen examples of decisions about undergoing diagnostic testing (particularly in Chapter 8), and nearly all medical decisions are informed by the results of tests.

Patients (and, indeed, many physicians), however, do not understand how diagnostic tests are developed or how to determine the value of the information they provide. The chapter case illustrates these concepts by examining the UBT for *H. pylori* infection, a relatively common diagnostic test for which there is a wealth of data about its effectiveness. In addition, diagnostic testing strategies involving multiple tests in series or parallel are considered. Finally, this chapter also discusses psychological heuristics associated with diagnosis and conditions under which such judgments are helpful or misleading.

Developing diagnostic tests

Suppose that we want to know if Jane has an active *H. pylori* infection without forcing her to undergo invasive endoscopic testing. Instead, we perform a UBT that measures change in the ratio of $^{13}CO_2$ to $^{12}CO_2$ (denoted by δ) exhaled by the patient 30 minutes after ingestion of ^{13}C-urea compared with the ratio before ingestion. Because *H. pylori* hydrolyzes ^{13}C-urea to $^{13}CO_2$, the resulting change value, $\Delta\delta$, tends to be higher in patients with *H. pylori* infection than the average uninfected patient, but there's natural variation both groups, and it's not impossible that a healthy patient could have a high $\Delta\delta$.

The situation is described graphically in Figure 10.1, adapted from Herold and Becker (2002). On average, infected patients have a higher $\Delta\delta$ than healthy patients, but the variation in each group is wide enough that we cannot easily categorize a patient with a $\Delta\delta$ of 6 as definitively healthy or infected.

The figure demonstrates the limits (and strengths) of the UBT's power to *discriminate* between the two groups. A more highly discriminative measure of infection results in a picture in which the curves of the two groups are more widely separated and have less overlap. A test that defines the disease (e.g., in the way that bacterial growth on a culture defines bacterial infection) and thus has, in principle, perfect discrimination, is often referred to as a "reference standard" or "gold standard" test.

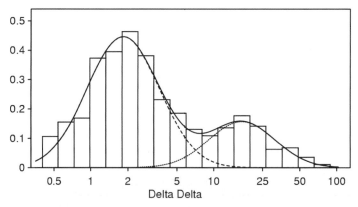

Figure 10.1 Distribution of $\Delta\delta$ for infected (bell curve on the right of the figure) and uninfected (bell curve on the left of the figure) patients. Both infected and uninfected patients may have $\Delta\delta$ as low as 3 or as high as 15. (Adapted from Figure 1 of Herold and Becker [2002], with permission of the BioMed Central Open Access license agreement; www.biomedcentral.com/info/authors/license).

Test thresholds

As $\Delta\delta$ gets higher, however, the person is more likely to be infected, and as it gets lower, they're more likely to be healthy. Our goal is to treat the sick differently than the healthy; for example, to prescribe a proton pump inhibitor and antibiotics if we are sufficiently convinced of the likelihood that the patient is, in fact, suffering from *H. pylori* infection. This implies that we need a criterion, or "threshold" $\Delta\delta$, above which we will act in one way (e.g., start drug therapy) and below which we will act in a different way (e.g., watch and wait). A threshold would be graphically represented by drawing a vertical line at the $\Delta\delta$ threshold score; patients whose $\Delta\delta$ is higher than the threshold are treated as infected, and those whose count is lower are treated as healthy. Such a threshold is shown in Figure 10.2.

As Figure 10.2 shows, because of the overlap between the distributions of $\Delta\delta$ (i.e., because of the imperfect discriminative power of $\Delta\delta$ in this example), no threshold can accurately classify every patient. Whatever criterion we set for calling someone infected or healthy based on this test, there will be some people rightly classified as infected or healthy, and some people wrongly classified as sick or healthy. For example, in Figure 10.2, the grey-shaded region represents infected patients with a $\Delta\delta$ higher than 5.78 who will be correctly classified as infected, and the black-shaded region represents noninfected patients with a $\Delta\delta$ higher than 5.78 who will be wrongly classified as infected.

The threshold determines the kind of error we are likely to make. The higher the $\Delta\delta$ threshold we require to call someone infected (graphically, the farther

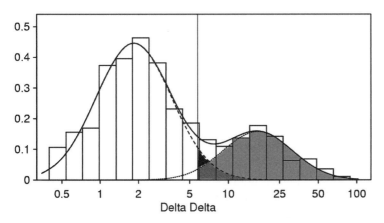

Figure 10.2 Impact of a threshold of $\Delta\delta = 5.78$ on classifying patients. (Adapted from Figure 1 of Herold and Becker [2002], with permission of the BioMed Central Open Access license agreement; www.biomedcentral.com/info/authors/license).

to the right we draw the vertical line), the more we'll wrongly classify infected people as healthy; these errors are called *false negatives*. For example, if we set the threshold at $\Delta\delta = 18$, we will almost never wrongly classify a healthy person, but about half of those infected will be misclassified as false negatives (and potentially remain untreated for their infection).

Conversely, the lower the $\Delta\delta$ we require, the more we'll wrongly classify healthy people as infected; these are *false positives*. For example, if we set the threshold at $\Delta\delta = 2$, we will almost never wrongly classify a infected person, but almost half of those not infected will be misclassified as false positives (and potentially undergo unnecessary treatment).

Changing the threshold will always either increase false positives and decrease false negatives or vice versa. Only improving the discriminative power can lower both false positives and false negatives.

Choosing thresholds

Unfortunately, we generally can't improve the discriminative power of a given test; we have to develop new and more discriminative tests (or variations of tests). But the choice of the threshold is arbitrary. A threshold may be recommended by the test developer or by guidelines on the use of the test. These thresholds should be chosen on the basis of the purpose of the test, and the consequences of false positives and false negatives.

For example, consider a rapid strep antibody test for strep throat. A false positive on this test results in a patient receiving an unnecessary dose of antibiotics for a few days; a false negative results in a patient with an untreated bacterial infection for a few days (until the results of the throat culture, a gold standard test, are available). The general consensus among physicians has been that a few days of unnecessary antibiotics is generally preferable to missing a bacterial infection for a few days, but not so preferable that antibiotics should be routinely started in all patients. Accordingly, the kits are developed to have a relatively low, but not very low, threshold for positive results. When the cost of a false negative is much greater, tests may have a very low threshold. A 17-year-old with unknown vaccination history who presents to the emergency department with high fever and neck stiffness is very likely to receive immediate presumptive treatment for meningitis. Although the probability of bacterial meningitis is quite low, the consequences of missing a case are so high that a marginally positive finding on a test with low discrimination (neck stiffness) is sufficient to warrant the relatively benign treatment pending culture results.

In general, when noninvasive and inexpensive tests are used to screen a population for a serious condition, the goal of testing is to broadly identify individuals who may be at higher risk for the condition and refer them for confirmatory testing or other evaluation. Screening tests, therefore, are usually designed to have very few false negatives and are willing to accept a larger number of false positives to ensure that high-risk cases are not missed.

On the other hand, when the treatment is invasive and the cost of the disease is low or when the primary aim of the test is to provide reassurance that a patient does not have a serious condition, false positives may be a much greater concern than false negatives. A high threshold is required of a test for carpal tunnel syndrome if the treatment contemplated is open carpal tunnel release surgery.

Sensitivity and specificity

Test developers and users are understandably reluctant to discuss their tests in terms of the number of false positives and false negatives that would be expected for a given threshold. Instead, test characteristics are usually reported as the test's *sensitivity* and *specificity*. This is akin to reporting how full a glass of water is rather than how empty.

Sensitivity is the rate of true positives; of patients who are in fact sick, what proportion does the test correctly diagnose? For example, a 95% sensitive test produces a positive result for 95% of sick patients who undergo the test. A moment's consideration reveals that the sensitivity is another way to speak about the rate of false negatives: if the test is positive in 95% of the sick patients, it is (falsely) negative in 5% of the sick patients. Accordingly, for screening tests and other situations in which false-negative results are particularly bad, highly sensitive tests are ideal.

Similarly, specificity is the rate of true negatives; of patients who are in fact healthy, what proportion does the test correctly diagnose? For example, a 90% specific test produces a negative result for 90% of healthy patients who undergo the test. Another moment's consideration reveals that the specificity is another way to speak about the rate of false positives: if the test is negative in 90% of the healthy patients, it is (falsely) positive in 10% of the sick patients. Accordingly, for confirmatory tests before invasive procedures and other situations in which false-positive results are particularly bad, highly specific tests are ideal.

For the UBT at 30 minutes, the sensitivity is 96%; that is, among a group of infected patients, 96% of them will have a positive UBT (the remaining 4% will be false negatives). The specificity of the test is also 96%; among a group of noninfected patients, 96% will have a negative UBT (the remaining 4% will be false positives; Herold and Becker, 2002)

The ROC curve

Recall that the balance of false positives and false negatives (and therefore sensitivity and specificity) depends on the discriminative power of the test (which we

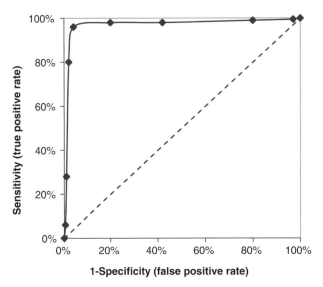

Figure 10.3 ROC curve for UBT at 30 minutes. (Drawn from data presented by Herold and Becker [2002]).

usually can't influence) and the threshold (which we can). For a given test, one can examine the impact of varying the threshold from low to high by plotting the resulting sensitivity and specificity or, more conventionally, the true positive rate (sensitivity) against the false positive rate (100% – the specificity). This kind of plot is called an "ROC curve."[1]

ROC curves can be used to compare the performance of different tests for the same condition. In general, more discriminative tests have ROC curves that bow out more strongly toward the upper left of the chart (more true positives and fewer false positives) and less discriminative tests have curves that approach the dotted diagonal line, which represents performance no better than chance (the same rate of true and false positives). The area under the ROC curve, which can vary from 0.5 to 1.0 square units, provides a numerical measure of the discriminative power of the test; it is generally equivalent to the proportion of patients (sick or healthy) that will be correctly classified (that is, the total percentage of true positives and negatives). For example, Figure 10.3 presents the ROC curve for the UBT, which correctly classifies 99% of patients. The $\Delta\delta = 5.78$ threshold is represented by the point in the upper left of the ROC curve, as it provides 96% sensitivity and 96% specificity.

---

[1] ROC stands for "receiver operating characteristic," which is such a mouthful that it's rarely used in conversation; ROC is instead pronounced "R-O-C." The term comes from signal detection theory and originally was used to describe the performance of radio receiver operators in World War II. See Green and Swets (1966).

Table 10.1 The CAGE questionnaire (Ewing, 1984)

Score one point for each question to which the patient answers "yes":	
C(ut):	Have you ever felt you should Cut down on your drinking?
A(nnoy):	Have people Annoyed you by criticizing your drinking?
G(uilty):	Have you ever felt bad or Guilty about your drinking?
E(ye-opener):	Have you ever had a drink first thing in the morning to steady your nerves or get rid of a hangover?

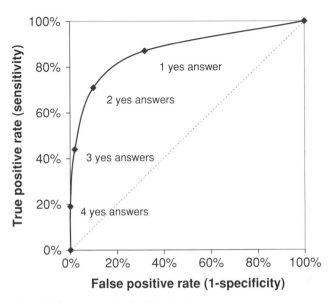

Figure 10.4 ROC curve for the CAGE test.

ROC curves can also be used to examine the properties of tests that have a small number of discrete scores, as well as those that use a threshold for a continuous score. For example, Table 10.1 shows the four-item CAGE questionnaire for alcoholism; one point is scored for each question answered affirmatively (Ewing, 1984). The threshold for further workup for alcoholism can be set at any number of affirmative answers, and Table 10.1 displays the ROC curve for different thresholds on the CAGE questionnaire (Sackett 1992; Schorling, 2005).

In the figure, it is clear that if a single "yes" answer is used as the threshold for further workup, the true positive rate is quite high (most alcoholics will be correctly referred), but the false positive rate is also reasonably high (over a quarter of nonalcoholics will be incorrectly referred for further workup). If two "yes" answers are required, the proportion of alcoholics identified drops to about 70%, but the number of false positives drops even more sharply, to about 10%. In fact, a threshold of two "yes" answers is generally recommended.

Interpreting diagnostic tests

In daily practice, of course, we do not develop new diagnostic tests. Instead, we select from available tests with recommended thresholds. The selection is based, ideally, on the characteristics of the test (sensitivity and specificity) and the decision that will be taken depending on the test result.

Patients are rarely interested in the sensitivity of a test – what proportion of sick people test positive. Their concern is the meaning of a positive (or negative) test to *them* – of those who test positive, what proportion are actually sick? The latter value is the "predicted probability of a positive test" or *positive predictive value,* and depends not only on the sensitivity and specificity of the test, but on the prior (before-testing) likelihood that the patient was sick. When a condition is rare, or the patient is unlikely to have the condition because of other clinical factors, the positive predictive value of a test for the condition will be lower than if the condition is prevalent or the patient has other factors that increase suspicion of the condition.

The difference between test characteristics and predicted values is easily illustrated with tests for smallpox. Polymerase chain reaction (PCR) tests for smallpox are very accurate; for example, assume that these tests have a sensitivity of 95% and a specificity of 99.99%. Of healthy people who are given such a test, only 0.01% (1 in 10 000) will have a false positive result. Consider a patient who presents to a physician with a rash and receives (among other tests) a smallpox test that has a positive result. Is the patient likely to have smallpox? The simple answer is "no." Because smallpox has been eradicated, any positive test *must* be a false positive, no matter how unlikely.[2]

A more familiar example is mammographic detection of breast cancer in a 40-year-old woman with no familial risk of breast cancer. The sensitivity of a first-time mammogram is 70% to 80% in these women; the specificity is about 95%. However, the probability that a positive test is a true positive in such a patient is about 4%; few young patients have cancer, and of those who do, few have sufficiently advanced cancer to be detectable by mammogram at this age (Humphrey *et al.*, 2002).

For a female adolescent presenting with iron-deficiency anemia, the prevalence of *H. pylori* infection has been estimated at about 33% (Cardenas, Mulla, and Ortiz, 2006)[3] Given a sensitivity and specificity of 96% for the UBT, the

[2] Strictly speaking, as of the time of this writing, there remained some stockpiles of smallpox virus in the hands of large governments, and one can imagine acts of war or terrorism that could once again lead to suspicion of smallpox. Given the success of these governments at protecting these stockpiles to date, however, the probability of this occurrence is likely much lower than even 1 in 10 000.

[3] Other studies have provided estimates of prevalence as high as 66% among female adolescent athletes, but these studies were performed on considerably smaller samples than the Cardenas *et al.* (2006) study.

positive predictive value is 92%. The negative predictive value – the probability that a patient with a negative test is actually infected – is only 2%.

Bayes' theorem

If we know, or can estimate, the patient's prior probability of a condition, and we know the sensitivity and specificity of a test, we can determine the predicted values mathematically, using an equation called *Bayes' theorem*. In practice, the simplest way to apply Bayes' theorem is to use a calculator on a website (Schwartz 2000) or PDA (Centre for Evidence-Based Medicine, 2004).

One can also apply Bayes' theorem quickly using Fagan's nomogram (Fagan, 1975), depicted in Figure 10.5. To use the nomogram, the test characteristics must be expressed as a *likelihood ratio*, rather than sensitivity and specificity. A likelihood ratio for a given test result is the likelihood that a patient with the test

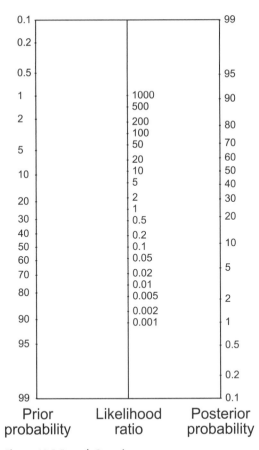

Figure 10.5 Fagan's Bayesian nomogram.

result would be from the sick rather than healthy population. For example, the likelihood ratio for a positive test (often abbreviated LR+) is the probability that a sick patient would have a (true) positive test (the test sensitivity) divided by the probability that a healthy patient would have a (false) positive test (100% − the test specificity). The likelihood ratio for a negative test (LR−) is the probability that a sick patient would have a (false) negative test (100% − the sensitivity) divided by the probability that a healthy patient would have a (true) negative test (the specificity). For the UBT, the LR+ is 96% ÷ (100% − 96%) = 24, and the LR− is (100% − 96%) ÷ 96% = 0.042.

An LR+ of 1 means that there are just as many true positives and false positives, so a positive result on the test gives no useful information; an LR− of 1 similarly means that a negative test is useless. Normally, the LR+ will be higher than 1 (a positive test result is more likely from the sick than healthy population) and the LR− will be a fraction lower than 1 (a negative test result is less likely from the sick than healthy population). An LR+ of 10 and an LR− of 1/10 represent the same relative power to rule in or rule out the condition.

After looking up or computing the likelihood ratio of the test result, Fagan's nomogram is used by projecting a straight line from the prior (pretest) proba- bility at the left of the nomogram, through the likelihood ratio at the center of the nomogram, and continuing the line until it reaches the right of the nomo- gram. The posterior (post-test) probability is then read off the right scale. For example, laying a ruler from 33% prior probability through a likelihood ratio of 24 yields a post-test probability of 92%. That is, if you believe a patient is 33% likely to have a condition (e.g., *H. pylori* infection) and they get a positive result on a diagnostic test for the condition with LR+ of 24 (e.g., UBT), you should now believe they are 92% likely to have the condition.[4] Figure 10.6 shows the nomogram with lines drawn through the likelihood ratios of 24 and 0.04 (the positive and negative likelihood ratios for the UBT).

Multiple tests

In some cases, a single diagnostic test may not be sufficient to warrant taking action. For example, if the treatment is invasive, and the test is imperfect, you may not be comfortable treating patients because the false positive rate is too high. In this situation, it is common to combine the results of multiple tests. Often the tests are chosen so that one has high sensitivity and the other has high specificity; together, the test results may serve to effectively rule in or rule out the condition.

When maximum accuracy is required, it may be necessary to apply the gold standard test after a less invasive test; for example, if ruling out *H. pylori* is critical, a negative result on the UBT (suggesting a 2% probability of infection)

---

[4] An interactive online version of the nomogram is available at http://araw.mede.uic.edu/cgi-bin/testcalc.pl.

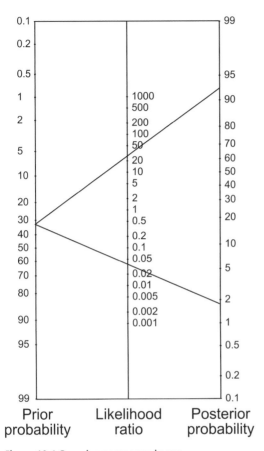

Figure 10.6 Bayesian nomogram in use.

may not provide enough comfort to forgo an endoscopy. On the other hand, a positive result on the UBT in that scenario would not require endoscopy. If endoscopy were necessary regardless of the UBT result, of course, it would be sensible not to perform the UBT test at all.[5]

Combining results

A good example of combining tests is blood testing for HIV infection. HIV testing typically includes a highly sensitive ELISA screening test paired with a highly specific Western blot test. Here's how the U.S. Preventative Services Task Force described the combination in 2005:

[5] Of course, in countries with a litigious culture, sometimes testing is undertaken for medicolegal reasons – to protect the physician, rather than the patient. It has been effectively argued that unnecessary "defensive testing" effectively transfers utility from patient to physician (or their insurer) and reduces the quality of patient care. See DeKay and Asch (1998).

A large study of HIV testing in 752 U.S. laboratories reported a sensitivity of 99.7% and specificity of 98.5% for enzyme immunoassay, and studies in U.S. blood donors reported specificities of 99.8% and greater than 99.99%. With confirmatory Western blot, the chance of a false-positive identification in a low-prevalence setting is about 1 in 250 000 (95% CI, 1 in 173 000 to 1 in 379 000).

(Chou *et al.*, 2005, p. 57)

Conditional independence

Although two tests are usually better than one, there is an important caveat about interpreting the result of multiple tests. Although it is appealing to begin with a patient's pre-test probability of disease, apply the first test to determine their post–first-test probability, and then use that updated probability as the prior probability for the second test, this strategy assumes that the test results are *conditionally independent* – that the likelihood ratio for a finding should not depend on the likelihood ratio for another finding. Put another way, two tests are conditionally independent if the people who are misclassified by the first test are not the same as the people who are misclassified by the second test.

For example, people who tend to be false positives on a single ELISA blood test for HIV are probably more likely to be false positives on a second ELISA. This means that positive results on two ELISAs is not going to increase the posterior probability as much as positive results on two independent tests. In fact, if ELISA is perfectly reliable, in the sense that someone who gets a false positive *always* gets a false positive, then the second "confirmatory" ELISA doesn't increase their likelihood of having HIV at all.

When research studies have been conducted that examine the use of two tests separately and in combination, reported likelihood ratios can be used to infer whether the tests are conditionally independent. If tests are conditionally independent, multiplying the likelihood ratios for the tests conducted separately should result in a likelihood ratio that is similar to the value for the tests combined. For example, in a study of UBT and an *H. pylori* stool antigen test (HpSA) in Egyptian children, Frenck *et al.* (2006) found that UBT had a positive likelihood ratio of 8.9 and the stool antigen test had a positive likelihood ratio of 3.0 – the product of these values is 26.7. In comparison, the positive likelihood ratio of a test strategy in which both tests were administered and patients were classified as positive or negative if both tests are positive or negative was 19.4, which is relatively similar to 26.7, suggesting the tests are largely conditionally independent. Unfortunately, nearly one-third of their patients received different test results on the UBT and HpSA, making the interpretation of this combination more difficult.[6]

[6] The authors of the study suggest that UBT's high negative predictive value suggests that a negative UBT may not require confirmation with HpSA and that the combined strategy might be most useful to confirm a positive UBT test noninvasively.

Strategies for ordering tests

Decision analysis has frequently been applied to compare alternative diagnostic workup strategies. For example, Gracia and Barnhart (2001) compared six strategies for diagnosing ectopic pregnancy in women presenting with abdominal pain or bleeding in their first trimester:

1. ultrasound followed by serum quantitative hCG
2. hCG followed by ultrasound
3. serum progesterone followed by ultrasound followed by hCG
4. progesterone followed by hCG followed by ultrasound
5. ultrasound followed by repeat ultrasound
6. clinical examination alone

Assuming that the primary goal was not to miss an ectopic pregnancy (that is, to have a low rate of false negatives), the study found that the first two strategies and the repeat ultrasound would maximize the sensitivity of the workup, detecting 100% of ectopic pregnancies. However, because the initial ultrasound is slightly better at ruling out ectopic pregnancy on its own than other initial tests, strategy 1 (ultrasound followed by serum hCG) would result in fewer false positives (leading to interrupted intrauterine pregnancies, some of which may have been viable) than the other two; its specificity was about 99%, whereas the others were about 98%.

Scoring rules

When a large number of potential indicators for a condition are available, conditional dependence may make it difficult to apply Bayes' theorem and develop appropriate likelihood ratios for each indicator. Instead, alternative mathematical techniques, based on regression, are often used to develop "clinical scoring rules."

A typical scoring rule assigns points to patient values on each indicator, provides an algorithm for combining the points (e.g., "add them up"), and then classifies patient risk or probability of disease on the basis of the range in which their score lies. That is, ranges of scores on the scoring rule are associated with likelihood ratios for the condition.

Two examples of prognostic scoring rules serve to illustrate their function and their usefulness. Kattan and colleagues (Kattan *et al.*, 1998; Kattan 2003) describe a nomogram that implements a scoring rule for the probability of a prostate cancer recurrence after prostatectomy. In this scoring rule, patient PSA value, clinical stage, and biopsy Gleason score are converted to points, added, and then transformed into a probability. Researchers studying this rule have found it to be generally accurate in its predictions and a useful tool for physicians (Greene *et al.*, 2004).[7]

---

[7] An interactive online version of the nomogram is available at www.nomograms.org.

Figure 10.7 illustrates a scoring rule developed at the Mayo Clinic for patients with type 2 diabetes (Christianson *et al.*, 2006). The rule predicts patient risk of coronary heart disease in the next 10 years on the basis of patient gender, age, years of diabetes, smoking history, hemoglobin A1c value, blood pressure, cholesterol levels, and microalbumin level. Such scoring rules can provide a rapid method of providing clinical insight into a patient's risk of disease or prognosis when there are many indicators or contributing factors.

When scoring rules are compiled into an electronic database, they can form the basis for a diagnostic decision support system (DSS). Such systems seek to provide the physician with additional diagnostic power by comparing a list of complaints, findings from history and physical examination, and clinical test values to a large set of potential diagnoses, and producing a complete differential diagnosis, with the probabilities of each candidate diagnosis. A recent review of diagnostic DSSs found several reports of significant beneficial effect of such systems on practitioner performance, but few studies reporting patient benefit (Garg *et al.*, 2005).[8] Although such systems have promise, patients have been shown to deem the diagnostic ability of physicians who consult a DSS to be inferior to those who do not (Arkes, Shaffer, and Medow, 2007). On the other hand, the same research team has found that jurors in malpractice cases may deem a physician more liable if the physician used a DSS and defied its recommendation, suggesting that laypeople may believe that a DSS improves diagnostic decision making (Arkes, Shaffer, and Medow, 2007).

The psychology of diagnostic testing

The key function of diagnostic testing is to enable us to revise our beliefs about the likelihood that a patient has a particular condition, and diagnostic tests are developed with particular characteristics that affect their ability to change beliefs. Bayes' theorem provides a formal method for quantifying the impact of a test result, but in practice, both patients and physicians tend to revise their beliefs intuitively, using judgmental heuristics.

Heuristic judgment is a consequence of the dual nature of the human judgment apparatus. Two distinct cognitive processes, often termed "intuition" and "reasoning," are enacted by two parallel cognitive systems, which psychologists refer to as System 1 and System 2, respectively. As Figure 10.8 illustrates, System 1 shares many features in common with perception – it is fast, automatic, and effortless and based primarily on associations between experiences. System 2, on the other hand, is slow, controlled, and governed by rules. Formal processes

---

[8] In contrast, other kinds of clinical DSSs, such as clinical reminders for prevention, disease management, and drug-dosing systems, had a considerably higher rate of studies displaying beneficial impacts.

Factors for assessing risk of CHD in next 10 years for patients with diabetes*

Female: Age (years)	<60	60 – 74.9	75 +
	0	9	22
Male: Age (years)	<60	60 – 74.9	75 +
	6	20	41
Diabetes duration (years)	<5	5 – 9.9	10 +
	0	2	5
Smoking status	Never	Former	Current
	0	0	2
HbA1c (%)	<7	7.0 - 7.9	8.0 +
	0	2	6
Systolic BP (mmHg)	<120	120-139	140 +
	0	1	4
Tot Cholesterol / HDL	<4	4.0 – 5.9	6.0 +
	0	6	10
Microalbumin (µg/min)	<30		30 +
	0	-	1

Total cholesterol

350
325
300
275
250
225
200
175
150
125

HDL cholesterol

20
30
40
50
60
70
80

10
8
7
6
5
4
3

Total ÷ HDL cholesterol

Total score 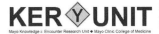 ___ + ___ + ___ = ___

Total score	Risk category**	Probability of having CHD in the next 10 years
00-17	Average	< 15%
18-31	Elevated	15 - 30%
32-69	High	> 30%

KER Ⓨ UNIT

Mayo Knowledge ↓ Encounter Research Unit ◆ Mayo Clinic College of Medicine

Based on the UKPDS Risk Engine and validated against 400 patients receiving diabetes care at Mayo Clinic Rochester. When calibrating this paper tool, we erred on the side of overestimation – this tool misclassifies approx. 5% of patients; note that it does not take into account family history of premature CHD or findings from noninvasive CV testing. The EVIDENS Research Group and the Knowledge and Encounter Research Unit prepared this aid thanks to grants from the American Diabetes Association. If you have questions, concerns or feedback **please** direct those to Victor Montori (Montori.victor@mayo.edu).

Figure 10.7 Coronary heart disease scoring rule for patients with type 2 diabetes (Christianson et al., 2006). Available online at: http://mayoresearch.mayo.edu/mayo/ research/ker_unit/decision-aids.cfm. Used with permission of the Mayo Foundation for Medical Education and Research ©Mayo Foundation.

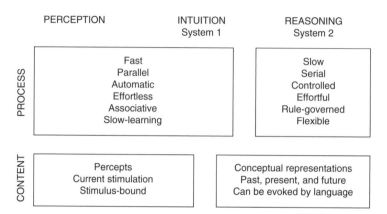

Figure 10.8 System 1 versus System 2. (Figure 1 from Kahneman [2003]. ©The Nobel Foundation [2002], with permission.)

for judgment, such as Bayes' theorem, rely on System 2 processing, and when no intuitive judgment is produced by System 1, System 2 is invoked.

In practice, however, an intuitive response from System 1 is often produced early in the judgment process and then is either (a) endorsed wholly by System 2, (b) used as an anchor for adjustments by System 2 based on other features of the task at hand, or (c) ruled incompatible with valid reasoning by System 2 and prevented from being overtly expressed[9] (Kahneman, 2003). For example, many physicians seem to automatically form judgments about patients' personalities and intelligence on the basis of their socioeconomics status (van Ryn and Burke, 2000); for some physicians, such judgments may later be ruled inappropriate by System 2 and effort made to discount them.

Two primary intuitive heuristics apply to probability revision, and several common biases in probability revision resulting from the use of these heuristics have been documented by psychologists. The first, anchoring and adjustment, suggests that we select an initial, or anchor, probability with System 1 and then apply System 2 to adjust our beliefs from the anchor (Tversky and Kahneman, 1974). However, the adjustment is frequently insufficient, which leads to "conservatism," one of the earliest cognitive biases identified (Edwards, 1968).

The availability heuristic, discussed in Chapter 5, also gives rise to biases in probability revision. Because important or particularly harmful outcomes are more salient, the value of an outcome may be confounded with its probability.

---

[9] Preventing an intuitive response from being overtly expressed does not, however, prevent it from impacting judgment. Incompatible responses may find more subtle expression through making the effort of judgment more difficult or interfering with metacognitions used to select appropriate rules and methods for making a judgment.

As a result, it is difficult for everyday judgment to keep separate accounts of the probability of a particular disease and the benefits that accrue from detecting it. Probability revision errors by physicians that are systematically linked to the perceived cost of mistakes demonstrate the difficulties experienced in separating assessments of probability from values (Wallsten 1981; Poses, Cebul, and Collins, 1985). In addition, information presented or acquired late in a workup tends to be more salient, and as a result, such information is given more weight than earlier information, regardless of its diagnostic value (Chapman, Bergus, and Elstein, 1996).

Other biases in test selection and interpretation have also been noted. In collecting data, there is a tendency to seek information that confirms a hypothesis rather than data that facilitate efficient testing of competing hypotheses. This tendency has been called "pseudodiagnosticity" (Kern and Doherty, 1982) or "confirmation bias" (Wolf, Gruppen, and Billi, 1985). Similarly, the most common error in interpreting findings is overinterpretation: data that should not support a particular hypothesis, and that might even suggest that a new alternative be considered, are interpreted as consistent with hypotheses already under consideration. The data best remembered tend to be those that support the hypotheses generated. Where findings are distorted in recall, it is generally in the direction of making the facts more consistent with typical clinical pictures (Elstein, Shulman, and Sprafka, 1978; Friedman *et al.*, 1998).

No universally effective methods for debiasing these judgmental tendencies have been developed; indeed, because they are so deeply rooted in our intuitive system, and because our intuitive system is essential to everyday operation, it seems unlikely that such methods could ever be developed. Instead, we must pay close attention to the learning environments in which medicine is taught and practiced to ensure that associations between, for example, symptoms and underlying diseases, are more likely to be made correctly.

In his book *Educating Intuition*, Hogarth (2001) draws attention to learning environments, distinguishing between those that are "kind" and facilitate learning appropriate associations and those that are "wicked" and obstruct the development of such associations. Kind environments are associated with relevant feedback, which provides the information necessary to learn correctly, and exacting costs of error, which provides the motivation to refine associations. Wicked environments provide irrelevant feedback and are lenient about error, which prevents the irrelevancies from coming to our attention and being remediated. Hogarth also suggests that some of the keys to effective use of our two modes of judgment include seeking appropriate feedback, imposing "circuit breakers" in our decision making to force us to stop and check System 1 reasoning with System 2, accepting the possibility of conflict, and more regularly applying the scientific method (observation, speculation, testing, and generalization) to our judgments.

Summary

Diagnosis is rightly considered one of the most important aspects of medical decision making. Diagnostic tests are developed to fit particular medical decisions; the choice of a test depends in large part on the goals of the diagnostician. Clinicians have a variety of measures by which the performance of a test may be assessed, and formal tools exist to use test results to help a clinician revise their beliefs in a patient's putative diagnosis. In the absence of formal methods (and even in their presence), a powerful system of intuition guides judgments and can be both improved and checked by formal reasoning.

Questions for clinical practice

- What is my goal in testing this patient? Is it more important to screen for a potential condition, to rule in a diagnosis or to rule out a diagnosis?
- What is my current level of suspicion that this patient has the diagnosis?
- Which tests are available that can meet my goals, and how powerful and useful are they when applied to patients like this one? Will my treatment plan change as a result of either a positive or negative test?
- If there is a significant possibility of false positives or false negatives, how can I best explain that to my patient and advise them on how to proceed through the workup?

Part V

Beyond the individual

Family matters

Introduction

Mr. P. is a 65-year-old man newly diagnosed with moderately differentiated clinically localized prostate cancer. He has been married to Mrs. P. for 38 years; they have two grown children. Mr. and Mrs. P. have come to consult you about whether he should undertake surgery, radiation treatment, or watchful waiting.

Ms. A. is a 50-year-old woman whose mother, age 75, has mid-stage Alzheimer's disease. Ms. A. has been progressively assuming greater caregiver responsibilities and feels that she will soon have to take sole responsibility for making decisions about her mother's care. She has come to you for advice about how to handle her new role.

This chapter explores two very different areas that represent intersections of family relationships with medical decision science. First, the case of Mr. P. considers how a patient's decisions might be affected by the impact of his or her health and quality of life on other family members. Second, the case of Ms. A. considers the ramifications of making decisions on behalf of another family member who is unable to do so for themselves.

Family utility

Nearly all of the prescriptive research and theory in medical decision making focuses on how patients should make decisions to maximize their health benefits or how payers and societies should make decisions to maximize the benefits they provide to patients within their budget. Patients are considered as individuals who receive direct benefits from their health care decisions. But some physicians have called attention to the fact that most people live within family units and need to be considered in this context (Schmidt, 1978). This has been more than a theoretical consideration; studies have documented that physicians identified as exemplary by their peers routinely discuss their patients' options within the context of family (Marvel, Doherty, and Weiner, 1998).

In fact, it is fairly easy to see that our patients' families are involved in patients' health care benefits in at least two ways. First, patients whose family relationships provide them with intrinsic value may get to enjoy this value longer and more fully if they improve their life expectancy and quality of life. Second, improving a patient's health or extending his life may increase the quality of life of other family members.

The impact of these family utility factors on treatment decisions is developed and illustrated for prostate cancer in an important recent paper by Anirban Basu and David Meltzer, two internists at the University of Chicago.[1] Their analysis is based on a decision model that found that the best treatment option, the option with the highest expected utility, can be related to a person's marital status (Meltzer, Basu, and Egleston, 2001).

Benefits to patients with families

When Mr. P. chooses whether to seek active treatment of his prostate cancer, he is faced with a choice between treatments (surgery and radiation) and watchful waiting. Each of the treatments may provide some benefit in life expectancy and may reduce the chance of progression to metastatic cancer with its concomitant reduction in quality of life. On the other hand, each of these treatments is associated with costs, meaning they increase the probability of quality-reducing side effects, notably impotence, incontinence, and bowel dysfunction.

If Mr. P. is happily married, his quality of life is enhanced by his marriage and family. As a result, when his life is extended, each life year he gains is a year at higher quality than he would experience if he were unmarried (or unhappily married).[2] In effect, because Mr. P. is happily married he gets more QALYs per each year of his life year.

This additional health benefit that accrues to Mr. P. by virtue of his family relationships should be included when examining the overall utility impact of his treatment choice from a *societal* perspective. That is, extending the lives of people with fulfilling family ties results in overall greater utility (as measured by QALYs) to society.[3] In Mr. and Mrs. P.'s family-level perspective, however,

---

[1] Meltzer is also an economist at the Harris School of Public Policy Studies at the University of Chicago. Because their work is nearly the only research on family utility in medicine, this section of the chapter extensively reviews and follows their article (Basu and Meltzer, 2005).

[2] In part, this result is specific to the focus on prostate cancer, which affects primarily older men. A 65-year-old man who is unmarried is likely to remain so. A treatment decision affecting a 25-year-old man, on the other hand, would have to consider the probability that the patient would marry in the future, and thus be subject to family-related utility adjustments.

[3] Or, similarly, encouraging people to form meaningful and quality-enhancing relationships with one another increase the health benefits that accrue to society as a result of health care interventions. Analysis from a societal perspective is discussed more fully in Chapter 12.

the pleasure he derives from his relationships should have no effect on his treatment decision, because he does not expect to alter his relationships during his treatment. That is, Mr. P. may gain more from a life-extending treatment than an unmarried man, but Mr. P., who remains married throughout his treatment, will not notice the difference. However, the best decision from Mr. and Mrs. P.'s perspective might be different from the decision that unmarried Mr. Z. might make, particularly if quality of life and length of life outcomes are traded off in the decision.

This family effect is an instance of a more general principle introduced in Chapter 4. As a patient's quality of life improves, the benefit of extending his or her life increases; similarly, as a patient's life expectancy improves, the benefit of improving his or her quality of life increases.

Benefits to families of patients

Mr. P.'s health state necessarily impacts the quality of Mrs. P.'s life. If Mr. and Mrs. P. are happily married, interventions that allow Mrs. P. to spend more time, or higher quality time, with Mr. P. increase her quality of life as well. On the other hand, interventions that result in a lower quality of life for Mr. P. may impair Mrs. P.'s happiness, either through emotional effects (such as anxiety and depression) or reduction in the quality of their interaction. For example, if Mr. P.'s treatment renders him impotent, Mrs. P.'s quality of life may be reduced both because she sympathizes with his emotional upset at the side effect and because she may find some previously pleasurable sexual activities less available. In addition, if cancer treatment significantly weakens Mr. P., then Mrs. P. will need to provide more personal care to make up for what Mr. P. can no longer do for himself.

These have been called "spillover effects" and they are largely unaccounted for in most decision analyses and cost-effectiveness studies. But it is clear from Basu and Meltzer's work that this effect can impact treatment choice from both a family and societal perspective. From Mr. and Mrs. P.'s perspective, spillover may make some treatments more attractive than others because the benefit to Mrs. P. may cause one treatment to stand out among the others. From a societal perspective, health care interventions may be more beneficial (and thus more cost effective) when they have positive expected impacts that spill over onto other family members.

According to Basu and Meltzer's (2005) analysis, if family spillover is not considered, then watchful waiting has the highest expected value. Surgery results in a net loss of 1.57 QALYs and radiation results in a net loss of 0.72 QALYs. But after considering spillover effects on Mrs. P., the option with the highest expected value can change. If the couple's quality of life increases by about 0.1 per year as a result of Mr. P.'s continued survival (net of side effects), surgery remains a losing proposition on average (with an expected net loss of 0.58 QALYs to the couple as compared with watchful waiting). Radiation, on the other hand, now becomes a reasonable choice and results in an additional 0.27 QALYs to the couple, as a result of Mr. P.'s additional benefit from continuing his married life and Mrs. P.'s additional benefit from Mr. P.'s continued life.

If Mr. P. were 85 years old, however, his expected survival would be considerably less. Not only would he and Mrs. P. receive less benefit from life gain, but the impact of the potential adverse side effects on Mrs. P.'s quality of life could actually result in negative spillover effects, making treatment even less preferable for a married man than an unmarried man. This analysis suggests that the effect of these spillover effects can be related to age; therefore, age is important when determining the treatment option with the highest expected value.

Costs to families of patients

Family status also has important ramifications on the cost of care to patients. Families with multiple wage earners may have more flexibility with respect to their medical care because of their increased resources to pay for care. Families in which family members can serve as caregivers without a loss of income to the family similarly have resources that act to decrease the cost of care.

On the other hand, larger families require more resources than smaller families. Patients with families who face large medical bills are reluctant to deprive their family of those resources while they're alive, or saddle them with debt should they die.

For most individuals, health is, if not priceless, much more highly valued than personal wealth. Choices between personal health and family welfare, however, are much more difficult. Physicians whose patients have others depending on them should be particularly attuned to these nonmedical goals.

Do patients already consider family impacts?

Basu and Meltzer's analysis is first and foremost prescriptive. They seek to describe methods by which decision analyses can incorporate family utility, and to illustrate cases in which impacts on family quality of life may result in different recommendations to the decision maker or policy maker. But their article also provides persuasive evidence that individual clinical decisions may already evince concern for family utility.

They examined data from the Surveillance Epidemiology and End Results (SEER) database, which collects data from tumor registries in the United States, together with Medicare data on health care claims for the SEER patients. They analyzed the treatment choices of 9 094 newly diagnosed prostate cancer patients aged 65 and older with nonmetastatic tumors.

As predicted by their prescriptive models, married patients were more likely than unmarried patients to choose treatment over watchful waiting at younger ages, but less likely to choose treatment over watchful waiting as they got older. This crossover is a particularly striking success for their predictions. Widowed and separated or divorced patients behaved like unmarried patients, making it unlikely that their result was due to some difference associated with being "marriageable" or "ever married."

Surrogate decision making

We now shift our focus from spillover effects and their influence on determining best treatment decisions to how health care decisions should be made when patients are unable to communicate their wishes. Although these two questions are related, the connection has not been well defined; the first comes out the world of economics and the second from the world of bioethics.

Physicians are accustomed to making recommendations for others; patients, however, face additional and often unfamiliar complexities when they find themselves in a position of "agency" – responsible for decisions that affect the health of a child, an aged parent, or an incapacitated spouse. How can physicians guide patients in these situations?

It is important to recognize that there is a continuum of decision competence. The ideal decision maker is a competent adult with informed insight into their condition and their options, the ability to communicate their wishes, and access to beneficent counsel from professionals in medicine, law, and so on. At the other end of the continuum are patients who are completely unable to communicate or interact with others. Arrayed in the middle are patients who can communicate but lack other features of the ideal decision maker, such as adult status, informed insight, or access to beneficent counsel. For example, in most societies, children are not accorded the legal capacity to make decisions about their health. Similarly, psychiatric patients and the mentally disabled may, in some cases, not be fully competent (in either the legal or common sense) to make decisions.

Ms. A.'s mother, with mid-stage Alzheimer's disease, is usually lucid, and still able to understand medical information and communicate her wishes with respect to her care. Ms. A. and her mother recognize, however, that eventually she may no longer be able to do so. They are beginning to plan for how decisions will be undertaken on her behalf at that point.

Can patients make decisions in advance?

A popular approach to the problem of incompetence in decision making is the advance directive in the form of a living will. A person, knowing that he may one day be a patient unable to communicate his wishes about his health care, may record these wishes in a document with the expectation that the instructions will be followed should he become incapacitated. Living will statutes giving legal force to these wishes have been enacted throughout the United States and in many other countries.

Unfortunately, living wills are problematic for several reasons outlined recently by an important and controversial article by Fagerlin and Schneider (2004), entitled "Enough: The Failure of the Living Will." They argue that living wills do not and cannot serve their stated purpose, because of "stubborn traits of human psychology and persistent features of social organization." The problem with living wills according to these authors is that:

- Most people do not write them, even among groups that would be expected to face the need to consider the possibility that they will be incapacitated and unable to direct their own care, such as chronically or terminally ill patients.
- People who do write them do not properly ensure that they are available when they are needed. In many cases, their physicians and surrogates are unable to find their living will documents.
- People cannot predict their future preferences accurately. This problem has already been discussed at length in earlier chapters.
- People cannot articulate their preferences clearly in writing. In addition to difficulties with health literacy and legal language, people often cannot anticipate the impact of new technologies and provide sufficiently broad directions to cover novel situations.
- Decision makers cannot interpret them the way patients would like. The more difficult it is to articulate preferences clearly, the most likely it is that those reading the living will may misunderstand or be unsure how to apply its more general instructions to a particular situation.

Fagerlin and Schneider are strong advocates of advanced directives and want these directives to have meaning when they are called upon. They recommend that patients forego living wills in favor of naming a health care proxy (sometimes referred to as providing a "durable power of attorney for health care"). That is, although patients may set down their preferences in writing, they do better to select and empower a trusted person to represent their desires, rather than rely on the writing alone.

Who makes decisions when the patient can't?

Although any other competent decision maker could, in principle, assume responsibility for directing the care of a patient who is unable to do so for herself, in practice there are two groups of potential surrogate decision makers for most patients: physicians and family members. And although physicians have unique advantages as health care decision makers by virtue of their knowledge and experience of medicine, patients often prefer family members for their knowledge and experience of the patient, her lifestyle, and her values.

As physicians Arnold and Kellum (2003) point out in a review of the moral justifications for surrogate decision making, there are several reasons to prefer family members as surrogates. As a procedural matter, when patients select family members as surrogates – as they often do – physicians who accord surrogate status to those family members are respecting the autonomy and choice of the patient. More substantively, family members ought to be better able, in principle, to speak "as if" they were the patient and to represent the patient's wishes because of their extensive interactions and close relationships with the patient.

In addition, society may value the family as decision makers quite apart from the specific decisions to be made. Family members are likely to be most strongly affected by the patient's health care (through the spillover effects mentioned in the first section of this chapter), and may bear a significant financial burden for the cost of the patient's care. Moreover, social policy may encourage the empowerment of families as social units as a moral good in itself (Arnold and Kellum, 2003).

Not all surrogate decision makers are family members, of course. Some patients have no family or are estranged from their family. Others believe that their family would be incapable of following their wishes or being objective about health care choice due to the strong (and perhaps incapacitating) emotions the family might experience when faced with a significant health care decision for a close relative. As a result, some patients do in fact select their physician or trusted friends as their health care proxy.

How should surrogate decisions be made?

When decisions are made by a surrogate, how should the decision maker approach the decisions? Ethicists have generally identified two major approaches to surrogate decision making: *substituted judgment* and the *best interest standard*.

In substituted judgment, the surrogate attempts to make the decision *as it would have been made by the patient*. That is, the surrogate tries to act as a substitute for the patient and an extension of the patient's will. The surrogate may do this by applying the patient's own decisions, made before their incapacitation, and expressed in a living will or through conversation with the surrogate. If the patient is facing a situation for which they have not given the surrogate specific instructions, the surrogate may apply substituted judgment by attempting to use their knowledge of the patient's goals, values, and preferences to determine how the patient would have made the decision had they been able to.

The best interest standard, in contrast, does not require the same degree of knowledge about the patient. Rather than determine what the patient would have done (as in substituted judgment), best interest judgments seek to determine which course of action would be in the best interest of the patient. Clearly, knowledge of the patient's goals is helpful in defining their best interest; if the patient devotes her life to music, her best interest is likely to favor choices that preserve her musical ability. As patients remain alive and incapacitated for longer periods, and as new medical interventions are developed or studied, it becomes increasingly difficult to make substituted judgments about options the patient could never have considered. In this situations, best interest often becomes the relevant standard.

A recent study of patients with dementia from Alzheimer disease and their families found that few families adopted a pure substituted judgment approach to their decision making. Most either used the best interest standard when making decisions or believed that the two standards would result in the same decisions for their family member (Hirschman, Kapo, and Karlawish, 2006).

Do surrogate judgments agree with patient judgments?

A mountain of evidence has accumulated that suggests that surrogates are far from perfect at predicting the decisions that patients prefer. A recent review of this research found that surrogate and patient decisions typically agree about 70% of the time; put another way, surrogates mistake the patients' decisions nearly one-third of the time (Shalowitz, Garrett-Mayer, and Wendler, 2006). Although surrogates were most accurate when making predictions in scenarios involving patients' current health states, even that level of accuracy reached only 79%; when making predictions in scenarios involving dementia or stroke, in contrast, accuracy levels are about 58%.

Most interesting in this research is that the approximately 70% level of agreement is surprisingly consistent; no methods have been shown to reliably increase the ability of surrogates to predict their patients' wishes. Notably, surrogates who engaged in more conversations with their principals around end-of-life decision making performed no better than surrogates who did not (Shalowitz, Garrett-Mayer, and Wendler, 2006). This was shown most strongly (and surprisingly) in the SUPPORT (Surrogates' Agreement with Patients' Resuscitation Preferences) trial (Marbella *et al.*, 1998). Patients and families in the intervention arm of this large randomized trial had extensive interaction with specially trained nurses. The key outcome was whether surrogates could accurately predict patients' preferences for do-not-resuscitate versus CPR orders.

Despite the powerful (and costly) intervention, agreement between patients and surrogates never exceeded 80% and was indistinguishable from agreement in the control arm of the trial. There was also no difference in agreement by whether the surrogate was the patient's spouse, child, parent, or sibling; when surrogates were none of these, however, agreement was lower (approximately 65%). Agreement was also somewhat lower for older patients than younger patients.[4]

Although imperfect, surrogate judgments appear to be the best available method for patients to assert their preferences when they are no longer able to make or express judgments for themselves.

A role for the physician

The tasks for physicians involved in their patients' family matters are complex. A patient may make decisions that the physician would not have made for herself. In this chapter, we see that this can occur even when the patient and his physician agree on how the risks and benefits play out on the personal level. In fact, the patient may be making a decision that does not seem optimal at the personal patient level but is nevertheless an optimal decision at the family level.

The physician is responsible for educating her patient about testing or treatment options including possible risks and benefits. As this chapter shows, in some cases these risks and benefits might well include potential harms or benefits to other family members as a result of the patients' health decision; in other cases, the physician may be responsible for educating the patient's surrogate decision maker rather than the patient himself.

Indeed, another important task for the physician may be helping patients decide how they want health care decisions to be made when they are not able to communicate their desires. Many patients will opt to manage this need for advanced directives by using living wills. However, available evidence suggests that it might be better if the patient names a health care proxy to make these decisions in real time instead of attempting to prospectively write out how they want these potential decisions to be handled.

Summary

Family members play important roles in medical decision making in several ways. In addition to serving as sources of information and support for patients, this chapter highlights two other important ramifications of family relationships. First, patient decisions may be influenced by their family structure, both because patients with happy families may receive more benefit from extending

---

[4] An earlier phase of the SUPPORT trial examined the agreement between patient preferences and their physicians' judgments of their preferences. Physicians performed better than surrogates when making predictions for patients who desired a DNR (60% agreement for physicians vs. 44% for surrogates). On the other hand, surrogates performed better when making predictions for patients who desired CPR (88% for surrogates vs. 77% for physicians.)

their lives than patients without satisfying relationships and because patients may desire to make decisions that benefit their families as well as themselves. Second, patients often look to their families to serve as surrogate decision makers when they are unable to make health decisions.

Questions for clinical practice

- How will my patient's health choices impact his or her family? Has my patient given this due consideration? Have I?
- How can I help my patients to have their wishes considered if they are incapacitated and unable to communicate or make decisions?
- What information do surrogate decision makers need to help them fulfill their role?

Public health

Introduction

You have recently adopted the recommendation of the Advisory Committee on Immunization Practices of the U.S. Centers for Disease Control and Prevention to vaccinate all children ages 12 to 23 months against hepatitis A. At an 18-month visit, one of your patient's parents asks you about it. "With the rising costs of health care, does it really make sense to give kids *another* shot? I understand polio and tetanus, but hepatitis A?"

In the United States, physicians have traditionally focused their attention on the clinical treatment of their patients with only secondary concern for matters of public health or the cost of medical care; the duty to the patient was primary. This focus has changed dramatically, however, in the last 20 years as concerns with rising health care expenditures have caused both physicians and laypeople to question not only whether good care is being provided but also at what cost.

In most countries outside the United States, physicians have always been responsible for the broader health of their societies (James *et al.*, 2005). Particularly when health care resources have been explicitly limited, either by scarcity or policy, physicians have been important advocates of the provision of cost-effective care.

This chapter introduces elements of decisions involving public health. First, it considers the problem of the aggregation of value: how should society place a value on health states that may be evaluated differently by different patients? Second, the chapter discusses direct and indirect costs and savings associated with medical care and briefly explains guidelines for the measurement of medical costs to society. Finally, the chapter combines the two by introducing cost-effectiveness analysis as a model for allocating a budget to public health programs and reviews the cost effectiveness of several kinds of public health and medical interventions in current use. The chapter case illustrates all of the concepts by presenting research on the cost effectiveness of routine hepatitis A vaccination for children in the United States.

The societal perspective

Public health decisions typically bring health benefits to people and generate health costs that are paid by people. Depending on which group(s) of people are considered in the decision, the impact of the choice can look very different. The answer to this question – whose benefits and whose costs will be considered? – is referred to as the "decision perspective."

Decision perspective determines which benefits and costs are considered germane to making the decision. This is particularly important when the costs are not fully borne by the beneficiaries. For example, taking the *individual patient* perspective in the United States, patients who are covered by health insurance or government financing programs rarely pay the full cost of their care. As a result, such patients have an incentive to obtain as much care as possible at discounted prices; indeed, they may even be willing to take additional health risks because they know they can rely on coverage (economists call such an incentive structure a "moral hazard"). Although the individual patient perspective is appropriate for a single patient making a decision, it clearly cannot be the basis for public health decision making in societies where health care costs are pooled.

Although individuals do not pay for the full cost of their health care, another possible perspective would be that of the "payer," for example, an insurance company, health maintenance organization, or government-funded health care program (e.g., Medicare). The payer perspective considers those costs incurred by the payer, and those health benefits received by all the people covered by the payer (i.e., by those people to whom the payer seeks to provide health care). This perspective is often adopted by insurance companies and health services seeking to decide whether offering a new treatment is worthwhile and affordable; because the payer is limited in what it can spend, and interested solely in the welfare of its covered participants, such a perspective properly incorporates the payer's concerns.[1] The payer perspective typically does not include the costs incurred by the patients in obtaining their care (e.g., co-payments or portions not covered by the payer).

From a true public health standpoint, however, the payer perspective focuses only on those patients covered by the payer (which may be a small subset of the public) and ignores other important components of medical costs that are borne by the public at large. For example, when illness prevents a sufferer from working at their job, society loses the benefit of the worker's productivity during the period of illness; this represents a cost to society that is not included in the payer perspective, unless the payer also happens to be the patient's employer.[2]

---

[1] This is particularly true when the payer has no profit motive; for-profit insurance companies have an additional (and sometime conflicting) interest in minimizing costs that may not be fully captured by this perspective.

[2] If the patient does not have paid sick leave, this cost may be incurred by the patient and accounted for in the patient perspective, of course.

Similarly, the payer perspective does not account for benefits that result from interventions funded by the payer but received by those not covered by the payer. In the case of vaccinations, this might occur due to herd immunity: the vaccine may provide health benefits even to the unvaccinated.

Accordingly, public health decisions are usually analyzed from the *societal perspective*, in which all costs incurred by society (e.g., by a nation) are considered, and benefits received by any member of the society are sought. This broad perspective ensures that decisions focus on the health of the society and reflect the resources of the society. It is in society's interest to provide as much health care as possible to the public at the lowest possible cost within the health care budget (which reflects the relative priority that a given society places on health care versus other social goods such as education, defense, etc.).

The aggregation of value

Adopting the societal perspective implies the need to be able to measure health benefits to society across a variety of possible health interventions. Several approaches have been used.

Health benefits in monetary units

An early approach to measuring benefit focused on assigning a monetary value to the health benefits. Aggregating benefits then becomes as simple as adding the monetary values. This approach characterizes "cost–benefit analysis," which weighs the costs of a program against the (monetary) value of its benefits.

Assigning monetary values to health benefits is not always straightforward, because health is not a market good. How much is it worth to shorten the duration of the flu by two days – as distinct from saving the cost of two days of flu (e.g., the cost of care, lost wages, etc.), which can be incorporated into the "cost" side of the analysis rather than the "benefit" side? Two major methods are used to determine the monetary value that people place on health benefits: observed spending behavior and contingent valuation.

When actual spending behavior can be observed, it can provide insight into a market value for a health benefit. For example, if there are several different products that promise relief from two days of flu symptoms at different prices, analysis of the purchase of these products might reveal the amount of money that people consider equally valuable to relief from two days of flu symptoms. Such an observation would not be perfect, however, as the products likely have other effects (side effects, inconvenience of taking the product) that may influence their prices, and people may or may not consider costs such as lost wages. Moreover, such observation opportunities are difficult to come by in most important cases, because, as alluded to earlier, few people pay the actual cost of their care. For example, there are likely to be few observations of patients paying the cost of their emergency room care for a broken shoulder.

When spending behavior cannot be observed, contingent valuation methods can be applied. In this approach, groups of people are surveyed and asked whether they would be willing to pay a given amount to receive a given benefit. For example, survey respondents might be asked if they would be willing to pay $50 to shorten the duration of flu symptoms by two days. These surveys, if well-constructed, have the advantage of providing direct monetary values for health benefits. Unfortunately, they are also subject to well-known biases, including both income effects (if you don't have $50, you can't be willing to pay $50) and lack of attention to income (people stating that they are willing to pay enormous amounts).[3] Moreover, some kinds of health benefits – such a saving the life of a child – strike people as immoral to assign a monetary value to; even if a respondent believes there is an appropriate value, he may be reluctant to say so.

Health benefits in health units

A second approach to measuring benefit is to use natural health units – lives saved, hepatitis cases prevented, life years added, and so on. This approach was termed "cost-effectiveness analysis" to indicate that benefits refer to the effectiveness (in health terms) of the intervention.

A clear advantage of using natural health units is that they can often be measured objectively, on the basis of epidemiological data or clinical research. They do not require people to assign subjective values to the benefit, and do not lead to moral concerns about placing a dollar value on health.

If health benefits were uniformly objective, for example, additional years of life, such aggregation would be a relatively simple process. A hypothetical intervention that provided, on average, three additional life years to each patient who needed it, and that would be needed by 10 000 patients per year, could be expected to produce 30 000 additional life years per year.

Unfortunately, the usefulness of cost-effectiveness analysis in natural health units is largely limited to decisions between alternative interventions for the same health problem, because natural health units are rarely commensurable across diseases. A public health program that results in 1 000 fewer cases of carpal tunnel syndrome per year is superior to one that results in only 100 fewer cases at the same cost, but how should it be compared to a program that results in one additional life year per year or a two-day decrease in flu symptoms for 100 000 people per year?

---

[3] An alternative measure, willingness-to-accept (WTA) asks people to indicate how much money they would require to forgo a benefit (or to compensate for a harm). In general, WTA estimates tend to be higher than willingness-to-pay (WTP) estimates, and possibly less reliable, and analysts who perform contingent valuation nearly always prefer WTP. For an excellent review of the issues, see Bayoumi (2004).

Health benefits in utility units

A third – and recommended – approach to measuring benefit is to use utility or quality-of-life units, typically quality-adjusted life years (QALYs).[4] This approach is a specific type of cost-effectiveness analysis that is formally termed "cost–utility analysis." Its advantages are that it measures important components of health (including quality of life) and that it uses commensurable units, which makes it possible to compare the benefits of interventions for different health problems.

On the other hand, the problem of aggregation of health benefits becomes much more complicated when health benefits include not only objective improvements but also impacts on utility or quality of life, which is subjective and varies from individual to individual for the same health state. Several methodological challenges must be faced to use measures like QALYs for public health decision making. Most important among these are whose utilities should be considered.

Because quality of life is subjective, assigning quality weights to health states often implies performing some sort of utility assessment on people to determine how they regard the quality of the health state. Techniques for individual utility assessments were reviewed in Chapters 2 and 3. A surprisingly difficult question is who should be asked to make these utility assessments – whose utilities should be incorporated into public health decisions? Arguments have been made for several different groups.

Patients who suffer from the health state being evaluated are a natural group to perform utility assessments upon, because they have the most relevant experience with the health state. Patients, however, are likely to place more weight on their illness or disability than on those experienced by others. At the extreme, if each group of patients considers their illness to be the most important for society to address, each group can rate their health state to be of extremely poor quality in an effort to cause more resources to be directed toward it. Experts in health (e.g., physicians who treat patients with particular health problems) may have similar conflicts of interest, as well as more difficulty, as surrogates, in accurately evaluating the impact of the health state.

Community members in general provide a representative sample of health states. Many will be healthy and have no particular incentive to bias their evaluation of a variety of health states to direct resources; those who are sick and may have such an incentive will appear in the population in proportion to the number affected by their illness and thus will receive appropriate weighting when their values are combined with the healthy. As discussed in Chapter 3, healthy respondents are likely to be poor at predicting the burden of illness. Despite this concern, the community population is generally recommended for most public health decision making.

---

[4] QALYs are discussed extensively in Chapter 4.

For example, a 2002 study of quality of life in patients with hepatitis A infections interviewed 181 U.S. citizens by mail. Respondents performed time trade-off utility assessments for a single hepatitis A health state described in nine paragraphs; the symptoms would typically last about 39 days, although could potentially lead to serious sequelae. They found, on average, that men were willing to trade off 25 life days to avoid this health state, and women were willing to trade off 14 life days (Jacobs, Moleski, and Meyerhof, 2002).

It can also be argued that taxpayers, rather than all community members, are the most appropriate group on which to assess utilities, as taxpayers provide the resources spent by the health care system. Accordingly, there are both moral reasons (those who provide the resources should have a voice in how the resources are used) and methodological reasons (taxpayers have an incentive to see that their taxes will be used to maximum benefit) for this suggestion. Taxpayer samples are generally not used, however, because many medical conditions disproportionately impact those in poverty and without access to good care. To further ignore or underweight the health needs of this population because they do not pay taxes would be to place them in double jeopardy; in most societies, social values preclude such an undertaking.

Measuring medical costs

Accounting for the cost of a medical intervention seems like it should be a simpler proposition than determining how to measure and aggregate benefits to quality and length of life. After all, costs already have a natural unit (dollars, or euros, or whatever the local currency is), are objective, and are usually written out or recorded. Surprisingly, measuring medical costs turns out to be quite difficult, for several reasons.

Costs and charges

When a patient or payer receives a bill from a health service provider, the bill does not list the cost of care, but the "charge" for care from the provider. These charges vary from provider to provider, and reflect not only differences in cost (e.g., the cost of nursing labor may vary from region to region) but also differences in such factors as profit levels and market demand for services (e.g., a provider located in an affluent and image-conscious city may charge more for cosmetic surgery than one located elsewhere, despite equivalent costs). Similarly, when a third-party payer (e.g., an insurance company) pays for care, it may not pay the cost of care or the charge for care, but some other scheduled amount negotiated between provider and payer; these negotiations undoubtedly include exogenous factors beyond simply the cost of care.

From a societal perspective, it is true costs that matter.[5] Decision analysts who wish to incorporate costs into analyses to make public health recommendations must either find ways to measure actual costs or, more frequently, must estimate the cost of care, either by using charges and applying a "cost-to-charge" ratio based on the overall charge level of the provider (e.g., costs are 62% of charges) or by conducting some form of "microcosting," in which individual activities in the provision of health care are assigned costs and the overall cost is computed by summing the microcosts.

Medical and nonmedical costs

The cost of a health care intervention includes more than simply the price of a drug, the cost of supplies, and the salaries of health care professionals. Although these medical costs constitutes the major portion of health care costs for many tests and treatments, nonmedical costs can be substantial and at times even more influential.

The most important nonmedical cost is often the cost of productivity loss experienced due to illness, either by the patient or by a family member who must serve as their caregiver. For example, when a parent must stay home from work to care for a sick child who cannot go to school, society incurs a productivity loss as result of losing the parent's work for the day.

A variety of costs related to illness or treatment can be important. For example, in considering routine hepatitis A vaccination in the United States, some of the important costs include the cost of caring for patients with hepatitis A infection and sequelae, productivity losses based on the expected wage of the patient or caretaker, the cost of disease surveillance and response, the cost of vaccination, and the cost of managing adverse events from vaccinations.

Discounting future costs

Some costs are incurred immediately; others will be incurred in the future. For example, a new treatment for HIV may require the patient to take expensive pharmaceuticals for many years and to undergo regular monitoring tests. Because money now is more valuable than money later (as reflected in capital markets), costs that will be paid in the future are discounted. Typically, discounting is performed at a constant annual rate of 3% to 5%.

One implication of discounting is that interventions that produce savings in the short term and costs in the long term become relatively attractive. Not

---

[5] When it is in the public interest to provide health services at cost universally, government can fix costs or set up its own health care system. Even where these steps are not taken, however, public health decision making generally seeks to avoid subsidizing market effects or profits to private companies.

paying for screening tests is an example of such a strategy. Naturally, such a short-sighted approach to budgeting will lead to disaster if the short-term savings are not properly kept in reserve so that they (and their earnings) will be available to make payments in the long term.

Another implication of discounting is that cost analyses performed at different times must standardize their monetary unit across time; this is also required by the impact of inflation and deflation. An intervention that cost $500 in 1950 might cost $3 500 in 2007.[6] Accordingly, the cost of public health interventions must be compared using the same year's currency, for example, 2005 dollars.

Future indirect medical costs

Most economists agree that it is important to consider the immediate medical and nonmedical costs of health care, as well as the (discounted) future medical costs associated with a health care intervention. Some economists also suggest that society should consider (discounted) future indirect medical (and other) costs that result from a health care intervention (Johannesson, Meltzer, and O'Conor, 1997; Meltzer, 1997).

To see why this suggestion is controversial, consider a new treatment that extends life expectancy by 5 years. Those 5 years will be experienced at the end of the recipient's life, at a time when she or he is retired (and therefore not producing net economic value to society) and at an age when health naturally begins to deteriorate. It is likely, therefore, that the recipient will incur additional medical costs during these 5 years. By extending the recipient's life, then, the very act of living longer increases costs to society – put starkly, it is cheaper for economically nonproductive people to die younger than older.

Proponents of including future indirect costs point out that while such an inclusion does make life-extending interventions *relatively* less cost-effective in the elderly and the chronically ill, it also makes quality enhancing interventions relatively more cost-effective. Those who disagree point out that although it may be sensible to account for all future costs from related or unrelated illness, it is only sensible if quality-of-life measures also include the value associated with future resource consumption (Nyman, 2004). It is unclear whether commonly used quality-of-life or utility measures may (implicitly) include these values (Gandjour, 2006; Nyman, 2006).

Cost-effectiveness

Cost-effectiveness analysis seeks to quantify the health value provided per dollar spent on a health care program or intervention. Two guiding principles underlie

---

[6] Assuming, of course, that an intervention from 1950 is still appropriate in 2007!

cost-effectiveness analysis: a budget ceiling and a utilitarian approach to the distribution of health benefits.

The practice of cost-effective medicine is sensible only when there is a limited health care budget – when there are fewer resources available than the potential demand. With unlimited funds for health care, we should simply provide every service that has been shown to be the least bit effective. Although there is a small group of very wealthy individuals and countries who may fall into this category, nearly all modern societies face a greater demand for health services than can be provided either by public or private funding.

Cost-effectiveness analysis itself is a tool that implies a simple utilitarian moral framework: provide as much overall health to a population as possible, given the budget constraints. So long as this is the public health goal, simple cost-effectiveness approaches are ideal for optimizing health care spending. In many cases, however, societies have more complex ethical frameworks that result in multiple conflicting public health goals. For example, many societies seek not only to maximize overall health to the population, but also to ensure that the health benefits are equitably distributed across the population, to ensure that emergency care is always available, or to prioritize health care for the sickest members of the population (the so-called rule of rescue). We will return to these other social values in Chapter 13.

The cost-effectiveness ratio

To maximize the health benefits that can be provided for a given budget (e.g., in dollars), we need to know the cost-effectiveness of each potential health program (test, treatment, educational program, etc.), and we need to fund the more cost-effective programs before the less cost-effective programs. The *cost-effectiveness ratio* (CER) is the ratio of cost to health benefit. For example, $100 000 per life saved, $20 000 per case of HIV prevented, $75 000 per life year, or $45 000 per QALY.

As discussed earlier, for public health decision making the effectiveness measure needs to be one that can be aggregated across the population and that is commensurable across different health programs. Accordingly, most cost-effectiveness analysis follows the recommendations of the Panel on Cost Effectiveness in Health and Medicine convened by the U.S. Public Health Service (Gold *et al.*, 1996) and uses dollars-per-QALY.

When each of the potential health programs is independent in its effects (i.e., the implementation of one program does not impact the cost-effectiveness of another program), the optimal combination of programs is found simply by ranking them in order from most cost-effective (least cost per QALY provided) to least and then funding them in order until the budget is exhausted.

In practice, however, funding "until the budget is exhausted" is rarely used, in part because health care agencies can be reluctant to obligate all of their funds

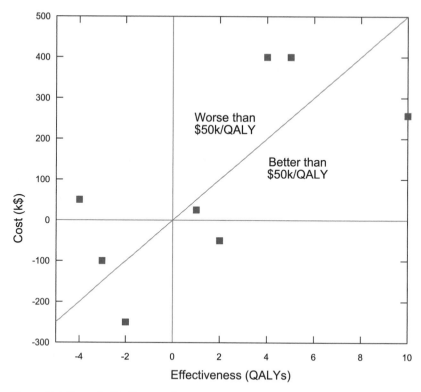

Figure 12.1 The cost-effectiveness plane.

at once, and in part because in many cases the budget ceiling is not precisely known. Instead, a threshold CER is identified; interventions that are less cost effective than the threshold are deemed "not cost-effective" and discouraged from funding.[7] This reflects the concept that societies might simply not be willing to pay $100 million dollars to gain one QALY. Typical thresholds currently in use are $50 000/QALY or $100 000/QALY.

Figure 12.1 plots a set of hypothetical health interventions on a cost-effectiveness plane. Effectiveness increases as points move from left to right; cost increases as points move from bottom to top. The diagonal line represents the $50 000/QALY threshold.

The upper right quadrant includes four programs that cost money and provide QALYs, like most medical treatments. Two programs are more cost-effective than the $50 000/QALY threshold: one provides 1 QALY per $25 000 spent,

---

[7] In practice, of course, few health care delivery systems are begun from nothing, and it is much more difficult to stop providing an existing benefit than to fail to cover a new benefit. As a result, many conventionally cost-ineffective procedures remain covered.

the other provides 10 QALYs per $250 000 spent. Two are less cost-effective, providing 4 or 5 QALYs per $400 000 (i.e., $100 000/QALY or $80 000/QALY respectively).

In the lower right quadrant are programs that are cost saving; they both provide health benefits and save money compared with the cost of not implementing the program. Preventative programs for widespread behaviors with serious health consequences, like smoking cessation programs, are often cost saving. The costs of the program can be dwarfed by the future savings in medical costs to the health care system, patient, or society.

Programs in the upper left quadrant both cost money and reduce health. These "cost-defective" programs should normally be ceased immediately when they are found to be detrimental to health. Frontal lobotomy for clinical depression is a historical example of such an intervention.

Programs in the lower left quadrant are problematic; these programs save health care dollars but reduce health benefits. For example, a hypothetical program that provides unhealthy fast food to visitors in hospital cafeterias (perhaps to use the savings to provide better televisions to hospital patients) falls into this quadrant. Some have argued that the cost-effectiveness framework itself results in rationing of health care to save money; that is, that all the currently provided effective interventions that society now considers too expensive to provide might also be considered in this quadrant.

Compared with no vaccination against hepatitis A, routine childhood vaccination at age 1 prevents over 172 000 hepatitis infections (and 32 deaths) in the cohort of 4 million children born in 2005. The resulting gain, 2 154 (discounted) QALYs, would be achieved at a cost of $60.9 million (including savings due to reducing productivity loss in patients and parents). The CER, therefore, is $28 000/QALY, making this a relatively cost-effective program (Rein *et al.*, 2007).

The incremental CER

The CER for an intervention compared with no intervention is sometimes called the "average" CER. It's a useful number when we can implement any combination of programs that we choose, and we're starting from scratch. More frequently, however, some programs are mutually exclusive or otherwise dependent on one another – for example, the cost or effectiveness of one smoking-cessation program may well depend on how many other such programs are already active in the milieu. In addition, programs are rarely compared against "no intervention"; often, there is already have some other standard of care in place.

In these cases, the statistic of interest is not the average CER but the "incremental" cost-effectiveness ratio (ICER): how much *more* health can a new intervention provide at how much *more* cost? To compute an ICER, divide the

Table 12.1 Sample ICERs from studies conducted in 2002–2003

Intervention vs. Comparison in Target Population	2002 $/QALY
Two intervention sessions on condom use alone VERSUS one control session on nutrition in non–HIV-infected urban women at high risk for STDs/HIV	$9,900
Six intervention sessions on sexual behavior and condom use VERSUS two intervention sessions on condom use alone in non–HIV-infected urban women at high risk for STDs/HIV	$140,000
Tamoxifen for primary prevention VERSUS no tamoxifen in women at very high risk of breast cancer (two or more first-degree relatives affected) – age 35	$45,000
Tamoxifen for primary prevention VERSUS no tamoxifen in women at very high risk of breast cancer (two or more first-degree relatives affected) – age 55	$89,000
Tamoxifen for primary prevention VERSUS no tamoxifen in women at very high risk of breast cancer (two or more first-degree relatives affected) – age 60	$140,000
Use of hip protectors VERSUS No use of hip protectors in women – age 65	Cost-saving
First-line therapy with ACE inhibitors VERSUS conventional first-line therapy with β-adrenoceptor antagonists or diuretics in male patients without cardiovascular comorbidity requiring antihypertensive drug therapy – age 40	$760,000

Data from the Center on the Evaluation of Value and Risk in Health.

incremental cost (how much more program B costs than A) by the incremental benefit (how many more QALYs program B provides than A).

Just as with average CERs, analysts often set a threshold ICER as a rule of thumb for cost-effectiveness; again, the most common thresholds are $50 000 (or pounds or euros) or $100 000 (additional) cost per (additional) QALY. An intervention might be cost-effective when compared with nothing, but quite cost-ineffective when compared to an existing standard of care that already provides most of the same benefits at a low price.

The CEA Registry of the Tufts-New England Medical Center's Center for the Evaluation of Value and Risk in Health provides a searchable database of cost-effectiveness analyses. It also provides several "league tables" listing the ICERs for a large number of interventions and comparisons. For example, Table 12.1 reproduces a small number of selected results from the database for analyses conducted in 2002 and 2003.

The examples in Table 12.1 illustrate several of the features of incremental cost-effectiveness analysis. The STDs/HIV intervention study shows that two intervention sessions can be quite cost-effective, but moving from two intervention sessions to six sessions is considerably less so. The tamoxifen study illustrates that the use of tamoxifen for primary prevention in high-risk women becomes less cost effective as the women get older (because older women are more likely to die from other causes of death, and thus receive less benefit). Finally, the hip protector study and ACE inhibitor study stand at opposite ends of the continuum of cost effectiveness; hip protectors actually result in cost savings (owing to reduction in costs of treating injury from falls), whereas first-line therapy with ACE inhibitors appears to be a costly approach to antihypertensive therapy in 40-year-old men without heart disease.

League tables regularly report only the CER, and the same ratio can be produced by interventions with very different impacts. For example, a program that provides 10 QALYs per patient for $100 000 per patient and could benefit 20 000 patients per year has the same ICER as a program that provides 0.1 QALYs per patient for $1 000 and could benefit 2 million patients per year. Cost-effectiveness analysis treats these programs as equally valuable, but policy makers might well have other reasons to favor one program over the other. This has led for some to call for "enhanced league tables" that provide additional information about the components of the ratio (Mauskopf, Rutten, and Schonfeld, 2003).

Compared with the standard vaccination levels against hepatitis A in the United States in 2003, routine childhood vaccination at age 1 would prevent over 112 000 hepatitis infections in the cohort of 4 million children born in 2005. The resulting gain, 1 240 (discounted) QALYs, would be achieved at a cost of $55.8 million (including savings due to reducing productivity loss in patients and parents). The ICER, therefore, is $45 000/QALY, making this a relatively cost-effective program (Rein et al., 2007). In fact, because of herd immunity, the actual benefit is probably greater – at no additional cost (Armstrong et al., 2007).

Arguments about cost-effectiveness

The use of cost-effectiveness in treatment decision making has not received uniform support among physicians. Indeed, the use of a public health perspective rather than an individual patient perspective is sometimes decried by physicians (particularly in developed nations) who see their sole duty as being to the welfare of whichever of their individual patients are under their care at any given time.

David Eddy's excellent book *Clinical Decision Making: From Theory to Practice* (Eddy, 1996) reviews and responds to many criticisms of cost-effectiveness analysis. Eddy presents 11 principles for making difficult decisions in difficult times. His principles focus on public health decision making but are addressed to physicians and form a framework for thinking about medicine as a social endeavor. They are:

1. The financial resources available to provide health care to a population are limited.
2. Because financial resources are limited, when deciding about the appropriate use of treatments it is both valid and important to consider the financial costs of the treatments.
3. Because financial resources are limited, it is necessary to set priorities.
4. A consequence of priority setting is that it will not be possible to cover from shared resources every treatment that might have some benefit.
5. The objective of health care is to maximize the health of the population served, subject to the available resources.
6. The priority a treatment should receive should not depend on whether the particular individuals who would receive the treatment are our personal patients.
7. Determining the priority of a treatment will require estimating the magnitudes of its benefits, harms, and costs.
8. To the greatest extent possible, estimates of benefits, harms, and costs should be based on empirical evidence.
9. Before it should be promoted for use, a treatment should satisfy three criteria: There should be convincing evidence . . . that the treatment is effective. Compared with no treatment, its beneficial effects on health outcomes should outweigh any harmful effects on health outcomes. Compared with the next best alternative treatment, the treatment should represent a good use of resources.
10. When making judgments about benefits, harms, and costs, to the greatest extent possible, the judgments should reflect the preferences of the individuals who will actually receive the treatments.
11. When determining whether a treatment satisfies the criteria of principle no. 9, the burden of proof should be on those who want to promote the use of the treatment (Eddy, 1996).

Although each of these principles has been challenged by opponents of cost-effectiveness analysis, the primary challenges fall into several basic lines.

First, physicians may feel that their professional ethics require that they have maximum autonomy to advocate for their patients over others. Even if it is important to consider public health, they may believe that it is not the role of the physician to consider resource allocation at the societal level. If patients agree with this concept of the physician's role, physicians who do not place their patients' welfare above others will garner distrust from their patients, who will be concerned that their physician is withholding an effective treatment because it is too costly. Similar concerns have been raised by patients in capitated health plans, in which primary care physicians receive a fixed yearly payment for each patient. In countries like Canada and the United Kingdom, where the need to ration health care resources is understood and accepted, these concerns are likely ameliorated by the knowledge that *every* physician is (ideally) applying a public health perspective.

Second, even if physicians consider public health to be an appropriate goal in their practice of medicine, there are methodological barriers to the acceptance of cost-effectiveness analysis as an approach to public health. Most physicians are not trained in cost-effectiveness analysis and may not be able to follow the analytic methods, but are asked to trust the results and apply them to their patients; this can be an uncomfortable position. In addition, good measurement of cost and benefit are difficult and can be demanding of data that are not always available in the clinical evidence base. These concerns have led to efforts to standardize cost-effectiveness analysis methods and to the formation of analytic centers within the U.S. Agency of Healthcare Research and Quality and the U.K. National Institute for Health and Clinical Excellence.

Finally, even when public health is an appropriate goal, and cost-effectiveness analysis in medicine is feasible, there are questions about whether cost-effectiveness alone is adequate to promote public health. In particular, societies may wish to express values, such as distributive fairness or constraints on acceptable medical procedures, that cannot be easily incorporated into CEA, in light of its utilitarian ethic (Brock, 2004). These social values are considered in depth in Chapter 13.

Summary

Physicians have an important role to play in advancing the health of the societies they serve. When health care resources are limited, clinicians and policy makers often look to cost-effectiveness analysis to help guide care decisions to maximize health provided to the public for a given level of resource expenditures. Cost-effectiveness analysis requires nuanced consideration of the measurement of effectiveness of health care across a population and the measurement of costs of health care; each of these has become a specialized field in itself. Although formally considering cost-effectiveness in care is not universally favored by physicians, cost-effectiveness analysis has the undisputed virtue of placing on the table issues of societal resource constraints and the need to truly understand the impact of new treatments.

Questions for clinical practice

- Who pays for the cost of my patient's care? Does the payer's budget require me to pay special attention to the cost-effectiveness of my health care recommendations?

- Given the care I'm already providing my patient, does it make sense to recommend different and more expensive approaches or stick with the current care plan?
- Are there interventions I can offer my patients which both save money in the future and improve health, such as preventative health care or lifestyle changes?

Social values

Introduction

> You and a colleague are discussing Praseedom *et al.*'s (2001) report of a 24-year-old patient whose cystic fibrosis progressed to end-stage lung disease and advanced liver disease, including cytomegalovirus infection. She weighs 52 kg and her FEV_1 is 0.8, which is only 25% of her predicted volume. She received a combined heart-lung-liver transplant, performed en bloc, and was treated with standard immunosuppression therapy for heart-lung transplant's recipients, along with perioperative prophylactic antibiotics for two days and nebulized colistin and tobramycin for one month. She survived for four months after the transplant, and then died from systemic cytomegalovirus infection.
>
> Aware of the scarcity of donor organs, you wonder aloud whether performing this multiorgan transplant was a good decision. Your colleague wonders how such a question could be answered.

Chapter 1 of this book began by considering the different types of goals that patients may use in making medical decisions and how physicians can assist their patients in clarifying their goals and selecting tests and treatments that will help their patients achieve their goals. This chapter once again takes up decision goals and objectives, but from the perspective of shared social values and ethical norms.

Ethics in clinical decisions

This book has approached medical decision making primarily from the standpoint of the community of clinicians, behavior scientists, and theorists who focus on the question of "how should decisions be made to provide the patient with the greatest health benefit?" Other groups of thinkers, including clinicians, philosophers, lawyers, and patient advocates, have asked an equally important question: "How should decisions be made to preserve the ethical values that mean most to us as individuals and societies?" Although decision scientists have traditionally emphasized utilitarian approaches to decision making, bioethicists have questioned whether one should focus on the consequences of decisions or their intrinsic features (as in deontological approaches to ethics). They have also asked such questions as whether morality is a feature of actions or a set of virtues, how moral claims should be justified, how to balance contextually specific decisions with universal principles, and how health care ethics relates to ethics in other endeavors (Khushf, 2004).

Like decision scientists, ethicists, particularly those who recognize multiple ethical principles, virtues, or rights, regularly consider situations in which all of their goals cannot be fully met. Decision science approaches this problem through prioritization and trade-off of goals. Ethics is more likely to use a process of "specification," in which each principle is made more contextual and concrete to provide guidance for the particular decision in question (Beauchamp and DeGrazia, 2004). Indeed, some philosophers advocate case-based approaches to bioethics, just as the judicial system in most Western nations interprets the law through the analysis of cases and the development of precedents (Boyle, 2004).

Although it would be natural to expect these two perspectives to converge and these two groups of theorists to share ideas, historically these questions have been answered through entirely separate academic endeavors and have resulted in separate communities of scholarship (Stiggelbout et al., 2006). Two recent studies have compared the thinking of decision scientists and bioethicists. In a survey by Ubel et al. (1996), 568 prospective jurors, 74 members of the American Association of Bioethics, and 73 members of the Society for Medical Decision Making were asked to choose between providing a more effective screening program to half a population (resulting in a greater number of deaths prevented overall) or a less effective program to the complete population (resulting in fewer deaths prevented overall). Decision scientists were less likely than others to favor the less effective (but arguably more equitable) program.[1]

A more extensive study by Stiggelbout et al. (2006) surveyed 327 members of the American Society for Bioethics and Humanities and 77 members of the Society for Medical Decision Making, presenting each participant with two clinical cases, one concerning refusal of a beneficial treatment and one concerning surrogate decision making about futile care at the end of life. The authors found substantial similarities in the opinions of the two groups, although decision scientists were more likely to emphasize outcomes and trade-offs and ethicists were more likely to emphasize patient autonomy. Notably, both groups called for greater exploration of patient goals and values, an ongoing theme of this book.

---

[1] Among all the groups, however, there was considerable variation. Fifty-six percent of jurors, 53% of ethicists, and 41% of decision scientists endorsed the less effective program.

As the Stiggelbout study suggests, the concerns of bioethics and decision science are often in alignment; the ethical principle of autonomy, for example, is often naturally reflected in the importance of properly eliciting and considering patient preferences in decision analysis. Bioethical principles can also be naturally incorporated into decision making as personal or societal constraints on possible choice alternatives: in a society that espouses the natural right of people to be free from becoming unwilling subjects of medical procedures, a decision alternative that results in forcing a family member to undergo genetic screening might be simply unacceptable. We alluded to such constraints in Chapter 1.

The remainder of this chapter considers two selected decision areas in which decision science and bioethics intersect, and each can enrich the other: rationing care in the context of limited resources and the conduct of medical research.

Rationing care

One of the primary ethical issues in medical care arises when it is not possible to provide unlimited care to all people, due to resource constraints. These constraints could take the form of a limited health care budget, as discussed in Chapter 12, but can also reflect limitations on the availability of facilities, equipment, personnel, or necessary treatments, including banked blood or donor organs. Bioethicists have described several different approaches to the problem of rationing care.

The utilitarian ideal

The utilitarian position seeks the greatest good for the greatest number, without regard to which individuals accrue benefit. Cost-effectiveness analysis (discussed in Chapter 12) embodies a utilitarian ideal of resource allocation.

Utilitarian approaches are favored in decision science but present several problems to the working clinician. First, clinicians have a long tradition of advocating for their own patients rather than for the patients of others. This advocacy is inherently at cross purposes with a utilitarian ideal and yet is extremely important both to physicians, for whom the art of medicine is most essentially practiced in the healing of the individual patient, and to patients, who wish to be assured that their physician is doing everything possible to heal them.

A second limitation of utilitarian rationing is that patients do not present simultaneously. The ability to make a optimal allocation that will achieve the greatest good for the greatest number is greatly challenged by the need to do so across a period of time. The utilitarian may be forced to withhold resources from patients present now to provide them, at greater benefit, to later patients who are absent in the moment. Failure to do so can reduce utilitarianism to a "first come, first served" ethic. On the other hand, too much withholding can lead to undertreatment of actual patients in the service of theoretical patients who may never materialize, and an overall reduction in benefit.

Nonmaleficence

Physicians are routinely reminded of their Hippocratic charge to "First, do no harm." The ethical principle of nonmaleficence expresses this duty by establishing a social taboo around initiating interventions that are intended or likely to cause direct harm to a patient or a group of people, even when such interventions may benefit others. For example, no matter how cost-effective a program of mandatory post-retirement euthanasia might be, and how many pre-retirement patients might benefit from improved care provided by the cost savings, such a program would not be ethically defensible. Nonmaleficence may appear to be a simple concept until one considers it is not always clear whether proceeding with a medical intervention or withholding the intervention is more harmful. Palliative care can be seen as conforming with this concept when further attempts at therapeutic intervention appear futile to the decision maker.

The rule of rescue

The rule of rescue charges the physician and the health care system to work hardest on behalf of those who are sickest and most in need of care, and particularly those whose lives are threatened (McKie and Richardson, 2003). This rule underlies the requirement of U.S. emergency departments to evaluate all patients who present with emergent needs, regardless of financial resources. The rule of rescue neatly avoids creating "double jeopardy" situations, in which those most in need of help have the least access to it. Researchers have found significant support for this ethic among the general population as well (Dolan, 2000).

The rule of rescue certainly does not optimize the use of health care resources. This rule results in high expenditures on hospital-based care instead of earlier, less costly, office-based care (Goldman, Joyce, and Zheng, 2007). In extreme cases, it justifies huge expenditures on patients who are very likely to die soon to achieve a small increment in the probability that they will survive a bit longer. This can be clearly seen in transplant cases. For example, patients with a failed heart transplant are often sicker than patients who need a transplant but have not yet received one. As a result, a new donor heart may be transplanted in the repeat transplant patient. But patients with a failed transplant are also much less likely to receive substantial benefit from a new transplant. The case of the 24-year-old cystic fibrosis patient presented at the start of this chapter is an even more extreme demonstration: the simultaneous transplantation of three organs (heart, lungs, liver) into a single patient rather than the distribution of the organs to three separate patients (Praseedom *et al.*, 2001; Murphy, 2002). The rule of rescue can thus lead to waste of donor organs, a scarce and limited resource.

In addition, the rule of rescue is often applied without sufficient regard for quality of life. A consequence of this kind of application is that life-saving and life-prolonging procedures are given very high social value, even when the cost of such interventions far outweighs their benefit to the patient. Although a finding of "medical futility" can limit the imperative to apply the rule of rescue, patients' interest in receiving as much care for themselves as possible can make such a finding difficult at best.

Triage

When personnel and supplies are limited, a norm of triage has also been applied, particularly in times of war or emergency. In triage medicine, patients with poor prognoses may receive only comfort care to preserve resources for patients with a better chance of survival. Among those patients who are deemed to have a chance to survive, preference is usually given to those in immediate need of life-saving treatment (like the rule of rescue), but sometimes given to those least injured (particularly among soldiers in war who are needed to return to the battlefield as soon as possible).

Equity

None of the preceding approaches to the ethics of care under limited resources broadly considers equity in treatment. Utilitarian approaches seek the greatest aggregate benefit without regard to how it is distributed, and the rule of rescue eschews equity in general for a narrow focus on the sickest patients. Considerations of equity in the rationing of health care demand attention to more features of how and to whom health care resources are allocated.

Procedural justice

Models of procedural justice seek to ensure that the process by which resources are allocated – the "how" – is fair. "Justice" here usually implies that every member of a population has an equal opportunity to receive care and equal access to that care when they need it.

When fewer resources are available than needed, procedural justice mandates that resources must be allocated through a method that does not allow any patient to gain an advantage over another patient through strategic means (by "gaming the system"). This tends to disfavor "first come, first served" approaches or decision-making approaches that rely on characteristics of individual patients. Instead, care may be rationed by lottery (in which all patients have an equal chance of receiving care or of moving to the head of a waiting list for care).

It has also sometimes been suggested that resources could be fairly allocated in proportion of the patient's objective contribution (or commitment to contribute) to the health care system. For example, if every citizen may choose to be an organ donor (or not), and choosing to do so has no financial cost, some have argued that those who agree to donate organs should thereby receive preferential status in the receipt of organs.

Providing preferential status in organ transplants to organ donors honors procedural equity. Many bioethicists argue, however, that providing any extrinsic reward to organ donors suggests that human organs (and, by extension, the human beings that provide them) may be treated as a commodity whose supply and demand are subject to the laws of the market. To paraphrase an old joke:

> A patient visits a doctor and asks him if he will perform a radical and unnecessary procedure on her for $10 million. He frowns, clearly uncomfortable, but in the end replies that for that kind of money, he'd be a fool not to. She then asks if he will perform it for $1. Offended, he asks, "What do you think I am?" She replies, "We've already established that you can be bought; now, we're just settling the price."

As the story suggests, bioethicists are concerned about a slippery slope from rewarding organ donation to wholesale commoditization of human tissue (Scheper-Hughes, 2003; Kahn and Delmonico, 2004), with particular concern about "medical tourism," in which affluent patients from developed nations travel to developing nations and purchase organ transplants from poor residents (Eighth Plenary Meeting of the Fifty-Seventh World Health Assembly in Geneva, 2005).[2]

In addition, a policy of preference transplant may implicitly devalue the decision to donate an organ in the first place. A robust finding in psychological research is that efforts that are motivated by an extrinsic reward are less well regarded, even by those exerting the effort, than those motivated by purely intrinsic considerations such as altruism (Deci, Koestner, and Ryan, 1999). Moreover, if the extrinsic reward is later removed, people become less likely to perform the effort than they were when no extrinsic reward was offered. Accordingly, preserving the status of organ donation as a purely charitable and altruistic gift may be important not only to avoid violating norms of the pricelessness of human beings but also to continue to encourage such donations and maximize overall societal utility.

Another procedural concern in organ donation involves the ability of donors to direct their organ donations to individuals. The United Network for Organ Sharing (UNOS) in the United States permits either nondirected donations

---

[2] Although some economists and philosophers have seriously suggested the creation of a market in organs. See, for example, Boudreaux (2006) and Radcliffe-Richards *et al.* (1998).

(which are provided to the next recipient-candidate on the waiting list) or donations directed to a particular named individual. Explicitly prohibited are donations directed to groups (e.g., to an unspecified person of a particular race, religion, or lifestyle), but such donations are becoming increasingly common nonetheless as "organ matchmaking" websites make it possible for potential donors to identify and name specific individuals who meet their group-based criteria (Murphy, 2006). Concerns about such practices by bioethicists who point out the need to balance justice and utility have led to calls to limit directed donation to family members (Zink *et al.*, 2005).

Distributive justice

In contrast to procedural justice, which concerns itself with how resources are allocated, distributive justice seeks to ensure equity among those to whom resources are allocated. That is, distributive justice is achieved when each member of the population receives his or her fair share of health care resources, regardless of the process by which this allocation occurs.

For example, theorists have discussed the so-called fair innings argument, in which health care should be provided to ensure that everyone receives at least a socially agreed upon sufficient length and quality of life (Williams, 1997). A consequence of this approach is that health care should be disproportionately provided to, for example, children, rather than adults, to increase their opportunities to experience their fair innings. This approach has also been compared with a pure "severity-based" approach akin to the rule of rescue in which those whose are worst off now or will be in the future should receive more health care resources (Nord, 2005).

Two of the major difficulties with the distributive justice ethic are determining what constitutes a "fair share" of resources and developing a process that ensures such a fair share. The former difficulty arises in part because the size of the resource pie to be divided, and the number of slices required, are often uncertain. In addition, some studies find people expressing a desire to distribute resources unfairly, to motivate or punish certain kinds of social behavior, such as treatment for those whose conditions may be related to their smoking, drinking, or diet behaviors (Shickle, 1997; Schwappach, 2002; Lenton, Blair, and Hastie, 2006). From a theoretical perspective, some philosophers have discussed ways to provide a limited but significant role to individual responsibility for health to balance the desire to motivate socially responsible choices with the desire to provide compassionate care to all (Cappelen and Norheim, 2006).

Social values and rationing care

Decision scientists and ethicists have noted that traditional cost-effectiveness analysis provides only for purely utilitarian decisions and have examined ways to modify the framework to incorporate not only utilitarian concerns but also additional social values (Menzel *et al.*, 1999). For example, Nord *et al.* (1999) considered three additional values: preference to provide care to those worst off (the rule of rescue), preference to provide care to those who will most benefit (a variation of triage), and preference to provide care that results in the greatest equality of health state among the population (distributive justice). Wagstaff (1991) reviewed similar concerns and discussed the possibility of a more general social welfare function that might be maximized rather than simply individual quality and quantity of life.

Ethics in medical research

Clinical research is a primary font of knowledge and evidence for medical diagnosis and treatment decisions. It would not be hyperbole to suggest that the (vast) medical research apparatus has made huge contributions to the quality, and sometimes affordability, of health care, particularly in the developed world. At the same time, clinical research engenders a host of ethical concerns beyond those of clinical care.

The guiding principles of ethical clinical research were established in the aftermath of the Nazi medical atrocities of World War II. The earliest of these principles, the requirement for voluntary consent, was enshrined in the Nuremberg Code of 1948 (on the history of which see Shuster [1997]). Later developments appear in the World Medical Association Declaration of Helsinki (Rickham, 1964) and, in the United States, in the Belmont Report of the National Commission for the Protection of Human Subjects (U.S. Department of Health, Education, and Welfare, 1979). The Belmont Report specifies three basic ethical principles: respect for persons, beneficence, and justice. At about the same time, the critically important book *Principles of Biomedical Ethics* put forward a very similar set of principles: respect for autonomy, nonmaleficence, beneficence, and justice (Beauchamp and Childress, 1979).

Respect for persons implies that research participation must be voluntary; all research subjects should be willing research subjects who freely choose to participate. This principle implies that subjects should not be coerced into participation, either through actual force, threat (to their persons, livelihoods, reputations, etc.), or disproportionate incentives. Another important implication of this principle is that potential subjects considering participation must have adequate knowledge of the research trial to make an informed decision about participation. As a result, the practice and process of *informed consent* has become one of key importance in the recruitment and participation of research subjects.

Beneficence is the principle that clinical research should be undertaken to provide benefit to society and in a manner that avoids harm to patients as much as possible (nonmaleficence). Research projects are regularly scrutinized by institutional review boards (IRBs) and funding agencies to ensure that the level of risk to which research subjects are exposed is commensurate with the level of benefit that the study may provide. Research that is known to lead to direct harm to human subjects should not, in general, be performed. Another important consequence of this principle is that placebo-controlled randomized clinical trials, in which subjects agree that they will be randomly assigned to receive a potentially beneficial treatment or a nonbeneficial placebo, should only be conducted when there is some doubt about the benefit of the treatment. Without such doubt (technically referred to in the ethics literature as "equipoise"), a placebo-controlled trial would effectively result in knowingly withholding a valuable treatment from a group of subjects.

Justice, discussed earlier in the context of rationing care, has particular application in research ethics. Notably, if a research trial involves risk to participants in the hope of yielding benefit, the potential benefit must also accrue to the participants, or those like them. A study in which one group is exposed to risk (at no benefit) to provide benefit (at no risk) to another group fails to meet the criterion of justice.[3]

Decision scientists have also considered medical research but have taken a different approach than have ethicists. Decision scientists are interested in the question of how best to allocate the available limited resources to competing research projects. A recent review of this question provides several methods for allocating scarce research resources: based on the burden of disease, the impact on clinical practice, or the value of the information which a trial is anticipated to generate (Fleurence and Torgerson, 2004). The authors argue that the best approach is the utilitarian one: allocation of resources such that research funding aligns with the goal of providing the most health benefits to the population.

Phase I drug trials

Phase I drug trials are conducted by pharmaceutical companies to establish the safe dose of a new pharmaceutical agent. Such trials typically proceed by exposing a relatively small number of subjects to different dosages of the agent and noting the relationship between dosage and toxicity. They are important because they facilitate the safe conduct of Phase II trials, which seek to measure the effectiveness of a drug in larger numbers of selected patients. Without Phase I trials, the development of new drugs would almost certainly result in greater harm to those treated with the drugs.

---

[3] The classic teaching example of injustice is the Tuskegee Syphilis Study, in which African-American men with syphilis were intentionally left uninformed of their disease and untreated, even when a proven cure was available. See, for example, Jones (1993).

Phase I drug trials are particularly troublesome with respect to research ethics. Two features of Phase I trials immediately stand out. First, many patients are likely to receive toxic overdoses during the Phase I process; the principle of nonmaleficence may not be met in the trial. Second, few patients are likely to receive clinical effective doses during the trial – if the agent is effective at all – so the overall beneficence of the trial is also low. Accordingly, such trials typically involve considerable risk at no benefit to the subjects enrolled to reduce the risk to subjects in later trials who may benefit from the drugs. This would seem to be a clear violation of standards of justice.

To justify such trials, therefore, participation is usually offered only to patients whose condition is so poor that there is no expectation of benefit with any alternative treatment, such as terminal cancer patients. For such patients, beneficence and justice may be less important considerations, as no treatment would be expected to provide benefit. Enrolling in a Phase I trial offers such patients no hope for improvement but does provide an opportunity to give additional meaning to their final days by altruistically contributing to future benefit for others.

This argument presupposes that patients who enroll in Phase I trials do so altruistically, and without unrealistic hopes of personal benefit. The informed consent process for such trials typically emphasizes the lack of expected benefit to the patient. Do participants in such trials actually understand the nature of the trial? Do participants in any medical research understand the nature of the study?

Informed consent

Unfortunately, research on the informed consent process suggests that research participants may not have good understanding. A major recent review of studies of informed consent comprehension in Phase I cancer trials found that fewer than half of patients understand the purpose of a Phase I trial, and a large group believe they will benefit from the trial (Cox, Fallowfield, and Jenkins, 2006). Moreover, participation decisions in clinical trials in general may be susceptible to relatively minor changes in the wording of consent forms (Schwartz and Hasnain, 2002). The order in which potential subjects learn about the risks and benefits of an intervention, a seemingly trivial consideration, may also influence whether an individual consents to a study (Bergus, Levin, and Elstein, 2002).

The requirements for effective informed consent for enrollment in a clinical research trial is an active area in bioethics, and one that is crucially important to physicians who seek to advise their patients on these decisions. There are several important ethical questions. Because human beings have cognitive limitations on the amount of information they can process, informed consent processes can present only a subset of the information available about the trial interventions without overwhelming patients – which subset should be selected? Which people are competent to provide consent? By what process should information be provided and consent obtained (and possibly documented)? Under what (emergency) conditions can treatment proceed without consent (Wear, 2004)?

Summary

Medical decisions do not occur in isolation from social values, and while decision scientific tools such as cost-effectiveness analysis may provide optimal recommendations to achieve important goals such as maximizing health benefit to a population, social norms, values, and ethics establish additional goals and constraints that are not as simply met. Clinical care, health care resource allocation, and medical research each present ethical concerns alongside their goals of providing care to patients, optimizing use of resources and maximizing information that will lead to improved care. Because no practical unified decision theory exists that incorporates all of the relevant social and individual values, clinicians must approach many decisions with concurrent attention to the outcomes of their patients and their ethical commitments.

Questions for clinical practice

- What are my ethical commitments to my patient, my profession, and my society? How might they be relevant to the decision I face?
- When health care resources that I use on my patient's behalf – including money, equipment, donor blood/tissue/organs, or my time – are limited, how should I distribute them ethically?
- When should I recommend enrollment in clinical trials to my patient?

Appendix: Summary of questions for clinical practice

Goals
- How deeply has my patient considered his/her goals?
- What does my patient want out of his/her life? What's important?
- How will treatment options impact my patient's ability to achieve his/her goals?
- Are there things my patient simply won't do out of strongly held conviction?

Dimensions of health
- Which dimensions of health are most important to my patient?
- How fully has my patient considered these dimensions?
- How do treatment alternatives differ in their impact on each dimension?

Overall health
- How can my patient best understand an overall health state?
- How can I help my patient anticipate what a future health state may be like?
- When do I need to measure or compare utilities for overall health states, and how should I do it?

Quantity and quality of life
- How will my patients' decisions impact their quality and quantity of life?
- Are my patients giving too much weight to short-term, transitory outcomes, at the expensive of their long-term health?
- How can I best illustrate the course of health that my patients can expect?

Uncertainty
- What are the most important uncertainties in the decision facing my patient?
- How does my patient regard risk and uncertainty in his or her life? Does she or he believe in taking chances to achieve big rewards or prefer to opt for smaller but surer results?
- How can I most effectively and accurately communicate the level of uncertainty associated with a diagnosis, a treatment, or a prognosis to my patient?
- How can I help my patient to cope with their lack of certainty about outcomes or options?

Choices and outcomes

- What are the expected, or average, outcomes that my patient will receive under each treatment option?
- Once a treatment option is selected, what are the actual outcomes that my patient should prepare for?
- If my patient does not use the expectation principle, how might she or he be making decisions? Could these approaches result in poorer outcomes?

Confidence

- When I provide patients with estimates, such the likelihood that their disease will progress or a treatment will be successful, would they benefit from knowing the statistical confidence interval around the estimate?
- When I provide patients with estimates, how (subjectively) confident am I in my estimate, and why?
- Are there opportunities to improve my confidence judgments (or those of my associates) by getting regular feedback about calibration or creating systems to ensure that disconfirming evidence will be considered?

Visualizing decisions

- Have my patients considered the sequences of choices they may face and constructed a list or map of strategies?
- How can I help my patients to consider the advantages and disadvantages of each of their potential strategies?
- Would a decision tree or influence diagram help my patients to better understand the clinical features of the decisions they face?

Information

- What uncertainties could change the decision if more information were available about them?
- What opportunities exist for gathering additional information? Is the cost of doing so worth the potential benefit?
- What sources of information are available from the clinical research literature?

Screening and testing

- What is my goal in testing this patient? Is it more important to screen for a potential condition, to rule in a diagnosis, or to rule out a diagnosis?
- What is my current level of suspicion that this patient has the diagnosis?
- Which tests are available that can meet my goals, and how powerful and useful are they when applied to patients like this one? Will my treatment plan change as a result of either a positive or negative test?
- If there is a significant possibility of false positives or false negatives, how can I best explain that to my patient and advise them on how to proceed through the workup?

Family decisions

- How will my patient's health choices impact his or her family? Has my patient given this due consideration? Have I?
- How can I help my patients to have their wishes considered if they are incapacitated and unable to communicate or make decisions?
- What information do surrogate decision makers need to help them fulfill their role?

Public health

- Who pays for the cost of my patient's care? Does the payer's budget require me to pay special attention to the cost-effectiveness of my health care recommendations?
- Given the care I'm already providing my patient, does it make sense to recommend different and more expensive approaches or stick with the current care plan?
- Are there interventions I can offer my patients which both save money in the future and improve health, such as preventative health care or lifestyle changes?

Social values

- What are my ethical commitments to my patient, my profession, and my society? How might they be relevant to the decision I face?
- When health care resources that I use on my patient's behalf – including money, equipment, donor blood/tissue/organs, or my time – are limited, how should I distribute them ethically?
- When should I recommend enrollment in clinical trials to my patient?

References

Ancker, J. S., Senathirajah, Y., Kukafka, R., *et al.* (2006). Design features of graphs in health risk communications: A systematic review. *Journal of the American Medical Informatics Association*, **13**(6), 608–18.

Antonopoulos, S. (2002). Third Report of the National Cholesterol Education Program (NCEP) Expert Panel on Detection, Evaluation, and Treatment of High Blood Cholesterol in Adults (Adult Treatment Panel III) final report. *Circulation*, **106**, 3143–421.

Arkes, H. R., Christensen, C., Lai, C., *et al.* (1987). Two methods of reducing overconfidence. *Organizational Behavior and Human Decision Processes*, **39**(1), 133–44.

Arkes, H. R., Shaffer, V. A., and Medow, M. A. (in press). The influence of a physician's use of a diagnostic decision aid on the malpractice verdicts of mock jurors. *Medical Decision Making*.

Arkes, H. R., Shaffer, V. A., and Medow, M. A. (2007). Patients derogate physicians who use a computer-assisted diagnostic aid. *Medical Decision Making*, **27**(2), 189–202.

Armstrong, G. L., Billah, K., Rein, D. B., *et al.* (2007). The economics of routine childhood hepatitis A immunization in the United States: The impact of herd immunity. *Pediatrics*, **119**(1), e22–9.

Armstrong, J. S. (2001). Combining forecasts. In *Principles of Forecasting: A Handbook for Researchers and Practitioners*. Dordrecht: Kluwer Academic, pp. 417–39.

Arnold, R. M., and Kellum, J. (2003). Moral justifications for surrogate decision making in the intensive care unit: Implications and limitations. *Critical Care Medicine*, **31**(5 Suppl), S347–53.

Asch, D. A., Baron, J., Hershey, J. C., *et al.* (1994). Omission bias and pertussis vaccination. *Medical Decision Making*, **14**(2), 118–23.

Baron, J., and Spranca, M. (1997). Protected values. *Organizational Behavior and Human Decision Processes*, **70**(1), 1–16.

Basu, A., and Meltzer, D. (2005). Implications of spillover effects within the family for medical cost-effectiveness analysis. *Journal of Health Economics*, **24**(4), 751–73.

Bayoumi, A. M. (2004). The measurement of contingent valuation for health economics. *PharmacoEconomics*, **22**(11), 691–700.

Beauchamp, T. L., and Childress, J. F. (1979). *Principles of Biomedical Ethics*. New York: Oxford University Press.

Beauchamp, T. L., and DeGrazia, D. (2004). Principles and principlism. In *Handbook of Bioethics: Taking Stock of the Field from a Philosophical Perspective*, ed. G. Khushf. Dordrecht: Kluwer Academic, pp. 55–74.

Bentham, J. (1970). *An Introduction to the Principles of Morals and Legislation (1789): The collected work of Jeremy Bentham.* London: Clarendon, p. 283.

Bergus, G. R., Levin, I. P., and Elstein, A. S. (2002). Presenting risks and benefits to patients: The effect of information order on decision making. *Journal of General Internal Medicine*, **17**(8), 612–17.

Bernoulli, D. (1954). Exposition of a new theory on the measurement of risk. *Econometrica*, **22**(1), 23–36.

Bier, V. M., and Connell, B. L. (1994). Ambiguity seeking in multi-attribute decisions: Effects of optimism and message framing. *Journal of Behavioral Decision Making*, **7**(3), 169–82.

Birnbaum, M. H., Patton, J. N., and Lott, M. K. (1999). Evidence against rank-dependent utility theories: Tests of cumulative independence, interval independence, stochastic dominance, and transitivity. *Organizational Behavior and Human Decision Processes*, **77**(1), 44–83.

Blais, A., and Weber, E. (2006). A domain-specific risk-taking (DOSPERT) scale for adult populations. *Judgment and Decision Making*, **1**(1), 33–47.

Bleichrodt, H., and Pinto, J. L. (2000). A parameter-free elicitation of the probability weighting function in medical decision analysis. *Management Science*, **46**(11), 1485–96.

Boudreaux, D. J. (2006). A free market in body organs. *Pittsburgh, PA: Pittsburgh Tribune-Review*, May 31, 2006. Retrieved March 3, 2007, from http://www.pittsburghlive.com/x/pittsburghtrib/opinion/columnists/boudreaux/s_456004.html

Boyle, J. (2004). Casuistry. In *Handbook of Bioethics: Taking Stock of the Field from a Philosophical Perspective*, ed. G. Khushf. Dordrecht: Kluwer Academic, pp. 75–88.

Brainerd, C., and Reyna, V. (1992). Fuzzy-trace theory: Some foundational issues. *Learning and Individual Differences*, **7**(2), 145–62.

Brase, G. L. (2002). Which statistical formats facilitate what decisions? The perception and influence of different statistical information formats. *Journal of Behavioral Decision Making*, 15(5), 381–401.

Brazier, J., Roberts, J., and Deverill, M. (2002). The estimation of a preference-based measure of health from the SF-36. *Journal of Health Economics*, **21**(2), 271–92.

Brazier, J. E., and Roberts, J. (2004). The estimation of a preference-based measure of health from the SF-12. *Medical Care*, **42**(9), 851–9.

Brewer, N. T., and Hallman, W. K. (2006). Subjective and objective risk as predictors of influenza vaccination during the vaccine shortage of 2004–2005. *Clinical Infectious Diseases*, **43**, 1379–86.

Brickman, P., Coates, D., and Janoff-Bulman, R. (1978). Lottery winners and accident victims: Is happiness relative? *Journal of Personality and Social Psychology*, **36**(8), 917–27.

Brock, D. (2004). Ethical issues in cost effectiveness analysis. In *Handbook of Bioethics: Taking Stock of the Field from a Philosophical Perspective*, ed. G. Khushf. Dordrecht: Kluwer Academic, pp. 353–80.

Brody, B. (2004). The ethics of controlled clinical trials. In *Handbook of Bioethics: Taking Stock of the Field from a Philosophical Perspective*, ed. G. Khushf. Dordrecht: Kluwer Academic, pp. 337–52.

Budescu, D., Karelitz, T., and Wallsten, T. (2003). Predicting the directionality of probability words from their membership functions. *Journal of Behavioral Decision Making*, **16**(3), 159–80.

Burstein, H. J., Gelber, S., Guadagnoli, E., *et al.* (1999). Use of alternative medicine by women with early-stage breast cancer. *New England Journal of Medicine*, **340**(22), 1733–9.

Bursztajn, H. J., Feinbloom, R. I., Hamm, R. M., *et al.* (1990). *Medical Choices, Medical Chances: How Patients, Families, and Physicians Can Cope with Uncertainty*. New York: Routledge.

Butcher, S. H. (1911). *Aristotle's Poetics*. London: Macmillan and Co.

Camerer, C., and Weber, M. (1992). Recent developments in modeling preferences: Uncertainty and ambiguity. *Journal of Risk and Uncertainty*, **5**(4), 325–70.

Cappelen, A. W., and Norheim, O. F. (2006). Responsibility, fairness and rationing in health care. *Health Policy*, **76**(3), 312–19.

Cardenas, V. M., Mulla, Z. D., Ortiz, M., *et al.* (2005). Iron deficiency and Helicobacter pylori infection in the United States. *American Journal of Epidemiology*, **163**(2), 127–34.

Cayley, W. (2004). I just want my pills. *Wisconsin Medical Journal*, **103**(2), 11.

Center for the Evaluation of Value and Risk in Health. (2007). The Cost-Effectiveness Analysis Registry. Boston: ICRHPS, Tufts Medical Center. Retrieved March 18, 2008 from www.cearegistry.org.

Centre for Evidence-Based Medicine. (2004). EBM calculator. University of Toronto. Retrieved March 18, 2008 from www.cebm.utoronto.ca/palm/ebmcalc/.

Chapman, G. B., Bergus, G. R., and Elstein, A. S. (1996). Order of information affects clinical judgment. *Journal of Behavioral Decision Making*, **9**(3), 201–11.

Chou, R., Huffman, L. H., Fu, R., *et al.* (2005). Screening for HIV: A review of the evidence for the U.S. Preventive Services Task Force. *Annals of Internal Medicine*, **143**(1), 55–73.

Choudhry, N. K., Anderson, G. M., Laupacis, A., *et al.* (2006). Impact of adverse events on prescribing warfarin in patients with atrial fibrillation: Matched pair analysis. *BMJ*, **332**(7534), 141–5.

Christianson, T. J. H., Bryant, S. C., Weymiller, A. J., *et al.* (2006). A pen-and-paper coronary risk estimator for office use with patients with type 2 diabetes. *Mayo Clinic Proceedings*, **81**(5), 632–6.

Claxton, K., Cohen, J. T., and Neumann, P. J. (2005). When is evidence sufficient? *Health Affairs*, **24**(1), 93–101.

Claxton, K., Sculpher, M., and Drummond, M. (2002). A rational framework for decision making by the National Institute For Clinical Excellence (NICE). *The Lancet*, **360**(9334), 711–15.

Claxton, K. P., and Sculpher, M. J. (2006). Using value of information analysis to prioritise health research: Some lessons from recent UK experience. *PharmacoEconomics*, **24**(11), 1055–68.

Constantine, N. A., and P. Jerman (2007). Acceptance of human papillomavirus vaccination among Californian parents of daughters: A representative statewide analysis. *Journal of Adolescent Health*, **40**(2), 108–15.

Cooke, A. D. J., and Mellers, B. A. (1998). Multiattribute judgment: Attribute spacing influences single attributes. *Journal of Experimental Psychology: Human Perception and Performance*, **24**(2), 496–504.

Cox, A. C., Fallowfield, L. J., and Jenkins, V. A. (2006). Communication and informed consent in phase 1 trials: A review of the literature. *Supportive Care in Cancer*, **14**(4), 303–9.

Cram, P., Fendrick, A. M. Inadomi, J., *et al.* (2003). The impact of a celebrity promotional campaign on the use of colon cancer screening: The Katie Couric effect. *Archives of Internal Medicine*, **163**(13),1601–5.

Damschroder, L. J., Zikmund-Fisher, B. J., and Ubel, P. A. (2005). The impact of considering adaptation in health state valuation. *Social Science & Medicine*, **61**(2), 267–77.

De Graves, S., and Aranda. S. (2005). When a child cannot be cured: Reflections of health professionals. *European Journal of Cancer Care*, **14**(2), 132–40.

Deci, E. L., Koestner, R., and Ryan, R. M. (1999). A meta-analytic review of experiments examining the effects of extrinsic rewards on intrinsic motivation. *Psychological Bulletin*, **125**(6), 627–68.

DeKay, M. L., and Asch, D. A. (1998). Is the defensive use of diagnostic tests good for patients, or bad? *Medical Decision Making*, **18**(1), 19.

De Wit, G. A., Busschbach, J. J., and De Charro, F. T. (2000). Sensitivity and perspective in the valuation of health status: Whose values count? *Health Economics*, **9**(2), 109–26.

Djulbegovic, B., Hozo, I., and Lyman, G. H. (2000). Linking evidence-based medicine therapeutic summary measures to clinical decision analysis. *Medscape General Medicine*, **13**, E6.

Dolan, J. G., Isselhardt, B. J., Jr., and Cappuccio, J. D. (1989). The analytic hierarchy process in medical decision making: A tutorial. *Medical Decision Making*, **9**(1), 40–50.

Dolan, P. (1996). Modelling valuations for health states: The effect of duration. *Health Policy*, **38**(3), 189–203.

Dolan, P. (2000). The measurement of health-related quality of life for use in resource allocation decisions in health care. *Handbook of Health Economics*, **1**, 1723–60.

Dolan, P., and Stalmeier, P. (2003). The validity of time trade-off values in calculating QALYs: Constant proportional time trade-off versus the proportional heuristic. *Journal of Health Economics*, **3**, 445–58.

Ebell, M. H., Bergus, G. R., Warbasse, L., *et al.* (1996). The inability of physicians to predict the outcome of in-hospital resuscitation. *Journal of General Internal Medicine*, **11**(1), 16–22.

Eddy, D. M. (1996). *Clinical Decision Making: From Theory to Practice, A Collection of Essays from JAMA*. Boston: Jones and Bartlett.

Edwards, W. (1954). The theory of decision making. *Psychological Bulletin*, **51**, 380–417.

Edwards, W. (1968). Conservatism in human information processing. In *Formal Representation of Human Judgment*, ed. B. Kleinmuntz. New York: John Wiley & Sons, pp. 17–52.

Edwards, W., and Barron, F. H. (1994). SMARTS and SMARTER: Improved simple methods for multiattribute utility measurement. *Organizational Behavior and Human Decision Processes*, **60**, 306–25.

Eichler, K., Puhan, M. A., Steurer, J., *et al.* (2007). Prediction of first coronary events with the Framingham score: A systematic review. *American Heart Journal*, **153**(5), 722–31.

Eighth Plenary Meeting of the Fifty-Seventh World Health Assembly in Geneva. (2005). Human organ and tissue transplantation. *Transplantation*, **79**(6), 635.

Elstein, A. S., Chapman, G. B., Chmiel, J. S., *et al.* (2004). Agreement between prostate cancer patients and their clinicians about utilities and attribute importance. *Health Expectations*, **7**(2), 115–25.

Elstein, A. S., Shulman, L. S., and Sprafka, S. A. (1978). *Medical Problem Solving: An Analysis of Clinical Reasoning*. Cambridge, MA: Harvard University Press.

Ewing, J. A. (1984). Detecting alcoholism: The CAGE questionnaire. *Journal of the American Medical Association*, **252**(14), 1905–7.

Expert Choice. (2004). *Expert Choice 11 [Computer software]*. Arlington, VA: Author.

Fagan, T. J. (1975). Letter: Nomogram for Bayes theorem. *New England Journal of Medicine*, **293**(5), 257.

Fagerlin, A., and Schneider, C. E. (2004). Enough: The failure of the living will. *The Hastings Center Report*, **34**(2), 30–43.

Feeny, D., Furlong, W., Boyle, M., *et al.* (1995). Multi-attribute health status classification systems: Health Utilities Index. *PharmacoEconomics*, **7**(6), 490–502.

Felli, J. C., and Hazen, G. B. (1998). Sensitivity analysis and the expected value of perfect information. *Medical Decision Making*, **18**(1), 95.

Fleurence, R. L., and Torgerson, D. J. (2004). Setting priorities for research. *Health Policy*, **69**(1), 1–10.

Florance, V. (1996). Clinical extracts of biomedical literature for patient-centered problem solving. *Bulletin of the Medical Library Association*, **84**, 375–85.

Fox, C. R., and Tversky, A. (1995). Ambiguity aversion and comparative ignorance. *The Quarterly Journal of Economics*, **110**(3), 585–603.

Fox, M., Mealing, S., Anderson, R., *et al.* (2006). *The effectiveness and cost-effectiveness of cardiac resynchronization (biventricular pacing) for heart failure: A systematic review and economic model*. London: National Institute for Health and Clinical Excellence.

Frenck, R. W., Jr., Fathy, H. M., Sherif, M., *et al.* (2006). Sensitivity and specificity of various tests for the diagnosis of Helicobacter pylori in Egyptian children. *Pediatrics*, **118**(4), 1195–202.

Friedman, C., Gatti, G., Elstein, A., *et al.*(2001). Are clinicians correct when they believe they are correct? Implications for medical decision support. *Medinfo*, **10**(Pt 1), 454–8.

Friedman, M. H., Connell, K. J., Olthoff, A. J., *et al.* (1998). Medical student errors in making a diagnosis. *Academic Medicine*, **73**(10), S19–21.

Froberg, D. G., and Kane, R. L. (1989). Methodology for measuring health-state preferences. II. Scaling methods. *Journal of Clinical Epidemiology*, **42**(5), 459–71.

Fryback, D. G., Dasbach, E. J., Klein, R., *et al.*(1993). The Beaver Dam Health Outcomes Study: Initial catalog of health-state quality factors. *Medical Decision Making*, **13**(2), 89–102.

Fryback, D. G., and Lawrence, W. F. (1997). Dollars may not buy as many QALYs as we think: A problem with defining quality-of-life adjustments. *Medical Decision Making*, **17**(3), 276.

Fryback, D. G., Lawrence, W. F., Martin, P. A., *et al.* (1997). Predicting quality of well-being scores from the SF-36: Results from the Beaver Dam Health Outcomes Study. *Medical Decision Making*, **17**(1), 1.

Gallant, M. P. (2003). The influence of social support on chronic illness self-management: A review and directions for research. *Health Education & Behavior*, **30**(2), 170–95.

Gandjour, A. (2006). Consumption costs and earnings during added years of life: A reply to Nyman. *Health Economics*, **15**(3), 315–17.

Garg, A. X., Adhikari, N. K. J., McDonald, H., *et al.* (2005). Effects of computerized clinical decision support systems on practitioner performance and patient outcomes: A systematic review. *Journal of the American Medical Association.* **293**(10), 1223–38.

Gigerenzer, G., and Hoffrage, U. (1995). How to improve Bayesian reasoning without instruction: Frequency formats. *Psychological Review*, **102**(4), 684–704.

Gigerenzer, G., and Selten, R. (2001). *Bounded Rationality: The Adaptive Toolbox.* Boston: MIT Press.

Gigerenzer, G., Swijtink, Z., Porter, T., *et al.* (1989). *The Empire of Chance.* Cambridge, MA: Cambridge University Press.

Gold, M. R., Siegel, J. E., Russell, L. B., *et al.*, eds. (1996). *Cost-Effectiveness in Health and Medicine.* New York: Oxford University Press.

Goldman, D. P., Joyce, G. F., and Zheng, Y. (2007). Prescription drug cost sharing: Associations with medication and medical utilization and spending and health. *Journal of the American Medical Association*, **298**(1), 61–9.

Government of Western Australia Department of Health. (2002). Consent form for radical prostatectomy. Retrieved March 3, 2008 from http://www.health.wa.gov.au/safetyandquality/programs/adult/urology/radical%20prostatectomy.pdf

Gracia, C. R., and Barnhart, K. T. (2001). Diagnosing ectopic pregnancy: Decision analysis comparing six strategies. *Obstetrics & Gynecology*, **97**(3), 464–70.

Green, D. M., and Swets, J. M. (1966). *Signal Detection Theory and Psychophysics.* New York: John Wiley & Sons.

Greene, K. L., Meng, M. V., Elkin, E. P., *et al.*(2004). Validation of the Kattan preoperative nomogram for prostate cancer recurrence using a community based cohort: Results from cancer of the prostate strategic urological research endeavor (CaPSURE). *Journal of Urology*, **171**(6 Pt 1), 2255–9.

Griffin, D., and Brenner, L. (2004). Perspectives on probability judgment calibration. *Blackwell Handbook of Judgment and Decision Making.* Oxford: Blackwell, pp. 177–99.

Groopman, J. E. (2007). *How Doctors Think.* Boston: Houghton Mifflin.

Grouzet, F. M., Kasser, T., Ahuvia, A., *et al.* (2005). The structure of goal contents across 15 cultures. *Journal of Personality and Social Psychology*, **89**(5), 800–16.

Harrison, J. D., Young, J. M., Butow, P., *et al.* (2005). Is it worth the risk? A systematic review of instruments that measure risk propensity for use in the health setting. *Social Science & Medicine*, **60**(6), 1385–96.

Haynes, R. B., McKibbon, K. A., Wilczynski, N. L., *et al.* (2005). Optimal search strategies for retrieving scientifically strong studies of treatment from Medline: Analytical survey. *BMJ*, **330**(7501), 1179.

Haynes, R. B., and Wilczynski, N. L. (2004). Optimal search strategies for retrieving scientifically strong studies of diagnosis from Medline: Analytical survey. *BMJ*, **328**(7447), 1040.

Herold, R., and Becker, M. (2002). 13C-urea breath test threshold calculation and evaluation for the detection of Helicobacter pylori infection in children. *BMC Gastroenterology*, **2**, 12.

Hershberger, P. J., Part, H. M., Markert, R. J., *et al.* (1994). Development of a test of cognitive bias in medical decision making. *Academic Medicine*, **69**(10), 839–42.

Hertwig, R., Barron, G., Weber, E. U., *et al.* (2004). Research article decisions from experience and the effect of rare events in risky choice. *Psychological Science*, **15**(8), 534.

Highhouse, S., and Hause, E. L. (1995). Missing information in selection: An application of the Einhorn-Hogarth ambiguity model. *Journal of Applied Psychology*, **80**(1), 86–93.

Hirschman, K. B., Kapo, J. M., and Karlawish, J. H. T. (2006). Why doesn't a family member of a person with advanced dementia use a substituted judgment when making a decision for that person? *American Journal of Geriatric Psychiatry*, **14**(8), 659.

Hogarth, R. M. (2001). *Educating Intuition*. Chicago: University of Chicago Press.

Hollon, M. F. (1999). Direct-to-consumer marketing of prescription drugs: Creating consumer demand. *Journal of the American Medical Association.* **281**(4), 382–4.

Howard, R. A. (1966). Information value theory. *IEEE Transactions on Systems Science and Cybernetics*, **2**(1), 22–6.

Humphrey, L. L., Helfand, M., Chan, B. K. S., *et al.* (2002). Breast cancer screening: A summary of the evidence for the U.S. Preventive Services Task Force. *Annals of Internal Medicine*, 137(5 Part 1), 347–60.

Hunink, M. G. M. (2005). Decision making in the face of uncertainty and resource constraints: Examples from trauma imaging. *Radiology*, **235**, 375–83.

Hux, J. E., and Naylor, C. D. (1995). Communicating the benefits of chronic preventive therapy: Does the format of efficacy data determine patients' acceptance of treatment? *Medical Decision Making*, **15**(2), 152–7.

Jacobs, R. J., Moleski, R. J., and Meyerhoff, A. S. (2002). Valuation of symptomatic hepatitis A in adults: Estimates based on time trade-off and willingness-to-pay measurement. *PharmacoEconomics*, **20**(11), 739–47.

James, C., Carrin, G., Savedoff, W., *et al.* (2005). Clarifying efficiency-equity tradeoffs through explicit criteria, with a focus on developing countries. *Health Care Analysis*, **13**(1), 33–51.

Johannesson, M. (1995). Quality-adjusted life-years versus healthy-years equivalents: A comment. *Journal of Health Economics*, **14**(1), 9–16.

Johannesson, M., Meltzer, D., and O'Conor, R. M. (1997). Incorporating future costs in medical cost-effectiveness analysis: Implications for the cost-effectiveness of the treatment of hypertension. *Medical Decision Making*, **17**(4), 382–9.

Jones, J. H. (1993). *Bad Blood: The Tuskegee Experiment*. New York: Free Press.

Kahn, J. P., and Delmonico, F. L. (2004). The consequences of public policy to buy and sell organs for transplantation. *American Journal of Transplantation*, **4**(2), 178–80.

Kahneman, D. (2003). Maps of bounded rationality: A perspective on intuitive judgment and choice. In *Les Prix Nobel. The Nobel Prizes 2002*, ed. T. Frangsmyr. Stockholm: Almqvist & Wiksell International.

Kahneman, D., Fredrickson, B. L., Schreiber, C. A., *et al.* (1993). When more pain is preferred to less: Adding a better end. *Psychological Science*, **4**(6), 401–5.

Kahneman, D., Slovic, P., and Tversky, A. (1982). *Judgment under Uncertainty: Heuristics and Biases*. New York: Cambridge University Press.

Kaplan, R. M., Bush, J. W., and Berry, C. C. (1976). Health status: Types of validity and the index of well-being. *Health Services Research*, **11**(4), 478–507.

Kareev, Y. (1992). Not that bad after all: Generation of random sequences. *Journal of Experimental Psychology: Human Perception and Performance*, **18**(4), 1189–94.

Kasser, T. (1996). Aspirations and well-being in a prison setting. *Journal of Applied Social Psychology*, **26**(15), 1367–77.

Kasser, T., and Ryan, R. M. (1993). A dark side of the American dream: Correlates of financial success as a central life aspiration. *Journal of Personality and Social Psychology*, **65**(2), 410–22.

Kasser, T., and Ryan, R. M. (1996). Further examining the American dream: Differential correlates of intrinsic and extrinsic goals. *Personality and Social Psychology Bulletin*, **22**(3), 280.

Kasser, T., and Ryan, R. M. (2001). Be careful what you wish for: Optimal functioning and the relative attainment of intrinsic and extrinsic goals. In *Life Goals and Well-Being: Towards a Positive Psychology of Human Striving*, eds. P. Schmuck and K. M. Sheldon. Cambridge: Hogrefe & Huber, pp. 116–31.

Kattan, M. W. (2003). Better predictions for patients. *Family Urology*, **8**(3), 11–15.

Kattan, M. W., Eastham, J. A., Stapleton, A. M., *et al.* (1998). A preoperative nomogram for disease recurrence following radical prostatectomy for prostate cancer. *Journal of the National Cancer Institute*, **90**(10), 766.

Katz, S., Ford, A. B., Moskowitz, R. W., *et al.* (1963). Studies of illness in the aged. The index of ADL: A standardized measure of biological and psychosocial function. *Journal of the American Medical Association*, **185**, 914–9.

Keeney, R. L., and Raiffa, H. (1976). *Decisions with multiple objectives: Preferences and value trade-offs.* New York: John Wiley & Sons.

Keller, S. D., Kosinski, M., and Ware, J. E. (1996). A 12-item short-form health survey (SF-12): A construction of scales and preliminary tests of reliability and validity. *Medical Care*, **32**(3), 220–3.

Kern, L., and Doherty, M. E. (1982). "Pseudodiagnosticity" in an idealized medical problem-solving environment. *Journal of Medical Education*, **57**(2), 100–4.

Khushf, G., ed. (2004). *Handbook of Bioethics: Taking Stock of the Field from a Philosophical Perspective*. Dordrecht: Kluwer Academic.

Kind, P. (1996). The EuroQoL instrument: An index of health-related quality of life. In *Quality of Life and PharmacoEconomics in Clinical Trials*, 2nd edn., Philadelphia, PA: Lippincott-Raven, pp. 191–201.

King, J. T., Jr, Styn M. M. A., and Tsevat, J. (2003). Perfect health versus disease free: The impact of anchor point choice on the measurement of preferences and the calculation of disease-specific disutilities. *Medical Decision Making*, **23**(3), 212–25.

Koehler, D. J., Brenner, L., and Griffin, D. (2002). The calibration of expert judgment: Heuristics and biases beyond the laboratory. In *Heuristics and Biases: The Psychology of Intuitive Judgment*, ed. T. Gilovich, D. W. Griffin and D. Kahneman. Cambridge, Cambridge University Press, pp. 489–509.

Koriat, A., Lichtenstein, S., and Fischhoff, B. (1980). Reasons for overconfidence. *Journal of Experimental Psychology: Human Learning and Memory*, **6**, 107–18.

Kramer, K. M., Bennett, C. L., Pickard, A. S., *et al.* (2005). Patient preferences in prostate cancer: A clinician's guide to understanding health utilities. *Clinical Prostate Cancer*, **4**(1), 15–23.

Kuhn, K. M. (1997). Communicating uncertainty: Framing effects on responses to vague probabilities. *Organizational Behavior and Human Decision Processes*, **71**(1), 55–83.

Lawton, M. P., and Brody, E. M. (1969). Assessment of older people: Self-maintaining and instrumental activities of daily living. *Gerontologist*, **9**, 179–86.

Lench, H. C., and Levine, L. J. (2005). Effects of fear on risk and control judgements and memory: Implications for health promotion messages. *Cognition & Emotion*, **19**(7), 1049–69.

Lenert, L. A., Sturley, A., and Watson, M. E. (2002). iMPACT3: Internet-Based Development and Administration of Utility Elicitation Protocols. *Medical Decision Making*, **22**(6), 464–74.

Lenton, A. P., Blair, I. V., and Hastie, R. (2006). The influence of social categories and patient responsibility on health care allocation decisions: Bias or fairness? *Basic and Applied Social Psychology*, **28**(1), 27–36.

Lerner, J. S., and Keltner, D. (2001). Fear, anger, and risk. *Journal of Personality and Social Psychology*, **81**(1), 146–59.

Levin, I. P., and Gaeth, G. J. (1988). How consumers are affected by the framing of attribute information before and after consuming the product. *The Journal of Consumer Research*, **15**(3), 374–8.

Lipkus, I. M., and Hollands, J. G. (1999). The visual communication of risk. *Monographs of the National Cancer Institute*, **25**, 149–63.

Lloyd-Jones, D. M., Wilson, P. W. F., Larson, M. L., *et al.* (2004). Framingham risk score and prediction of lifetime risk for coronary heart disease. *The American Journal of Cardiology*, **94**(1), 20–4.

Luce, R. D., and Fishburn, P. C. (1991). Rank-and sign-dependent linear utility models for finite first-order gambles. *Journal of Risk and Uncertainty*, **4**(1), 29–59.

Maddigan, S. L., Feeny, D. H., and Johnson J. A. (2004). Construct validity of the RAND-12 and Health Utilities Index Mark 2 and 3 in type 2 diabetes. *Quality of Life Research*, **13**(2), 435–48.

Maikranz, J. M., Steele, R. G., Dreyer, M. L., *et al.* (2006). The relationship of hope and illness-related uncertainty to emotional adjustment and adherence among pediatric renal and liver transplant recipients. *Journal of Pediatric Psychology*, **32**(5), 571–81.

Marbella, A. M., Desbiens, N. A., Mueller-Rizner, N., *et al.* (1998). Surrogates' agreement with patients' resuscitation preferences: Effect of age, relationship, and SUPPORT intervention. Study to understand prognoses and preferences for outcomes and risks of treatment. *Journal of Critical Care*, **13**(3), 140–5.

Marvel, M. K., Doherty, W. J., and Weiner, E. (1998). Medical interviewing by exemplary family physicians. *Journal of Family Practice*, **47**(5), 343–8.

Mauskopf, J., Rutten, F., and Schonfeld, W. (2003). Cost-effectiveness league tables: Valuable guidance for decision makers? *PharmacoEconomics*, **21**(14), 991.

McKie, J., and Richardson, J. (2003). The rule of rescue. *Social Science & Medicine*, **56**(12), 2407–19.

McNeil, B. J., Pauker, S. G., Sox, H. C., *et al.* (1982). On the elicitation of preferences for alternative therapies. *New England Journal of Medicine*, **306**(21),1259 –62.

Mehrez, A., and Gafni, A. (1989). Quality-adjusted life years, utility theory, and healthy-years equivalents. *Medical Decision Making*, **9**(2), 142–9.

Mellers, B. A. (2000). Choice and the relative pleasure of consequences. *Psychological Bulletin*, **126**(6), 910–24.

Meltzer, D. (1997). Accounting for future costs in medical cost-effectiveness analysis. *Journal of Health Economics*, **16**(1), 33–64.

Meltzer, D. (2001). Addressing uncertainty in medical cost-effectiveness analysis: Implications of expected utility maximization for methods to perform sensitivity analysis and the use of cost-effectiveness analysis to set priorities for medical research. *Journal of Health Economics*, **20**(1), 109–29.

Meltzer, D., Basu, A., and Egleston, B. (2001). Early results from a prostate cancer decision model. *Medical Decision Making*, **21**, 517.

Menzel, P., Gold, M. R., Nord, E., *et al.* (1999). Toward a broader view of values in cost-effectiveness analysis in health. *Hastings Center Report*, **29**(3), 7–15.

Mintzes, B., Barer, M. L., Kravitz, R. L., *et al.* (2002). Influence of direct to consumer pharmaceutical advertising and patients' requests on prescribing decisions: Two site cross sectional survey. *BMJ*, **324**(7332), 278–9.

Miyamoto, J. (2000). Utility assessment under expected utility and rank dependent utility assumptions. In *Decision Making in Health Care: Theory, Psychology, and Applications*, ed. G. B. Chapman and F. Sonnenberg. New York: Cambridge University Press, pp. 65–109.

Miyamoto, J. M., Wakker, P. P., Bleichrodt, H., *et al.* (1998). The zero-condition: A simplifying assumption in QALY measurement and multiattribute utility. *Management Science*, **44**(6), 839–49.

Mookadam, F., and Arthur, H. M. (2004). Social support and its relationship to morbidity and mortality after acute myocardial infarction: Systematic overview. *Archives of Internal Medicine*, **164**(14), 1514–18.

Murphy, A. H., and Winkler, R. L. (1982). Subjective probabilistic tornado forecasts: Some experimental results. *Monthly Weather Review*, **110**(9), 1288–97.

Murphy, A. H., and Winkler, R. L. (1984). Probability forecasting in meterology. *Journal of the American Statistical Association*, **79**(387), 489–500.

Murphy, T. F. (2002). The ethics of multiple vital organ transplants. *Hastings Center Report*, **32**(2), 47–8.

Murphy, T. F. (2006). Would my story get me a kidney? *Hastings Center Report*, **36**(2), 49–49.

National Safety Council. (2003). *Odds of dying*. Retrieved January 3, 2005, from http://www.nsc.org/lrs/statinfo/odds.htm.

Nease, R. F. (1997). Use of influence diagrams to structure medical decisions. *Medical Decision Making*, **17**(3), 263.

Nord, E. (2005). Concerns for the worse off: Fair innings versus severity. *Social Science & Medicine*, **60**(2), 257–63.

Nord, E., Pinto, J. L., Richardson, J., *et al.* (1999). Incorporating societal concerns for fairness in numerical valuations of health programmes. *Health Economics*, **8**(1), 25–39.

Nunes, T., Schliemann, A. D., and Carraher, D. W. (1993). *Street Mathematics and School Mathematics*. Cambridge: Cambridge University Press.

Nyman, J. A. (2004). Should the consumption of survivors be included as a cost in cost-utility analysis? *Health Economics*, **13**(5), 417–27.

Nyman, J. A. (2006). More on survival consumption costs in cost-utility analysis. *Health Economics*, **15**(3), 319–22.

O'Connor, A. M., Jacobsen, M. J., and Stacey, D. (2006). *Ottawa Personal Decision Guide*. Retrieved August 5, 2007, from http://decisionaid.ohri.ca/decguide.html.

Owens, D. K., Shachter, R. D., and Nease, R. F. (1997). Representation and analysis of medical decision problems with influence diagrams. *Medical Decision Making*, **17**(3), 241.

Parducci, A. (1965). Category judgment: A range-frequency model. *Psychological Review*, **72**(6), 407–18.

Parducci, A., and Perrett, L. F. (1971). Category rating scales: Effects of relative spacing and frequency of stimulus values. *Journal of Experimental Psychology*, **89**, 427–52.

Patrick, D. L., and Deyo, R. A. (1989). Generic and disease-specific measures in assessing health status and quality of life. *Medical Care*, **27**(3 Suppl), S217–32.

Paulos, J. A. (1988). *Innumeracy: Mathematical Illiteracy and Its Consequences*. New York: Hill and Wang.

Paulos, J. A. (1991). *Beyond Innumeracy*. New York: Knopf.

Peters, E., McCaul, K. D., Stefanek, M., *et al.* (2006). A heuristics approach to understanding cancer risk perception: Contributions from judgment and decision-making research. *Annals of Behavioral Medicine*, **31**(1), 45–52.

Poses, R. M., Cebul, R. D., Collins, M., *et al.* (1985). The accuracy of experienced physicians' probability estimates for patients with sore throats: Implications for decision making. *Journal of the American Medical Association*, **254**(7), 925–9.

Praseedom, R. K., McNeil, K. D., Watson, C. J. E., *et al.* (2001). Combined transplantation of the heart, lung, and liver. *The Lancet*, **358**(9284), 812–13.

Prosser, L. A., and Wittenberg, E. (2007). Do risk attitudes differ across domains and respondent types? *Medical Decision Making*, **27**(3), 281–7.

Radcliffe-Richards, J., Daar, A. S., Guttmann, R. D., *et al.* (1998). The case for allowing kidney sales. *The Lancet*, **351**(9120), 1950–2.

Redelmeier, D. A., and Kahneman, D. (1996). Patients' memories of painful medical treatments: Real-time and retrospective evaluations of two minimally invasive procedures. *Pain*, **66**(1), 3–8.

Redelmeier, D. A., Katz, J., and Kahneman, D. (2003). Memories of colonoscopy: A randomized trial. *Pain*, **104**(1–2), 187–94.

Redelmeier, D. A., Koehler, D. J., Liberman, V., *et al.* (1995). Probability judgment in medicine: Discounting unspecified possibilities. *Medical Decision Making*, **15**(3), 227.

Rein, D. B., Hicks, K. A., Wirth, K. E., *et al.* (2007). Cost-effectiveness of routine childhood vaccination for hepatitis A in the United States. *Pediatrics*, **119**(1), e12–21.

Reyna, V. F. (2004). How people make decisions that involve risk: A dual-processes approach. *Current Directions in Psychological Science*, **13**(2), 60–6.

Reyna, V. F., and Adam, M. B. (2003). Fuzzy-trace theory, risk communication, and product labeling in sexually transmitted diseases. *Risk Analysis*, **23**(2), 325–42.

Reyna, V. F., and Lloyd, F. J. (2006). Physician decision making and cardiac risk: Effects of knowledge, risk perception, risk tolerance, and fuzzy processing. *Journal of Experimental Psychology: Applied*, **12**(3), 179–95.

Rickham, P. P. (1964). Human experimentation. Code of ethics of the World Medical Association. Declaration of Helsinki. *British Medical Journal*, **5402**, 177.

Ritov, I., and Baron, J. (1990). Reluctance to vaccinate: Omission bias and ambiguity. *Journal of Behavioral Decision Making*, **3**(4), 263–77.

Rottenstreich, Y., and Tversky, A. (1997). Unpacking, repacking, and anchoring: Advances in support theory. *Psychological Review*, **104**(2), 406–15.

Saaty, T. L. (1980). *The Analytic Hierarchy Process: Planning, Priority Setting, Resource Allocation*. London: McGraw-Hill.

Saaty, T. L., and Vargas, L. G. (2001). *Models, Methods, Concepts & Applications of the Analytic Hierarchy Process*. Boston: Kluwer Academic.

Sackett, D. L. (1992). The rational clinical examination: A primer on the precision and accuracy of the clinical examination. *Journal of the American Medical Association*, **267**(19), 2638–44.

Sandman, P. M., Weinstein, N. D., and Miller, P. (1994). High risk or low: How location on a risk ladder affects perceived risk. *Risk Analysis*, **14**(1), 35–45.

Savage, L. J. (1954). *The Foundations of Statistics*. New York: Dover.

Scheper-Hughes, N. (2003). Keeping an eye on the global traffic in human organs. *The Lancet*, **361**(9369), 1645–8.

Schmidt, D. D. (1978). The family as the unit of medical care. *Journal of Family Practice*, **7**(2), 303–13.

Schorling, J. B. (2005). Review: Sensitivity of the CAGE questionnaire for the DSM diagnosis of alcohol abuse and dependence in general clinical populations was 71% at cut points> = 2. *BMJ*, **10**(1), 26.

Schwappach, D. L. B. (2002). Resource allocation, social values and the QALY: A review of the debate and empirical evidence. *Health Expectations*, **5**(3), 210–22.

Schwartz, A. (2000). *Diagnostic test calculator*. Retrieved March 3, 2008, from http://araw.mede.uic.edu/cgi-bin/testcalc.pl.

Schwartz, A., and Hasnain, M. (2002). Risk perception and risk attitude in informed consent. *Risk, Decision, and Policy*, **7**, 121–30.

Schwartz, A., Hazen, G., Leifer, A., *et al.* (in press). Life goals and health decisions—What will people live (or die) for? *Medical Decision Making*.

Schwartz, J. A., and Chapman, G. B. (1999). Are more options always better?: The attraction effect in physicians' decisions about medications. *Medical Decision Making*, **19**(3), 315.

Sevdalis, N., and Harvey, N. (2006). Predicting preferences: A neglected aspect of shared decision-making. *Health Expectations*, **9**, 245.

Shalowitz, D. I., Garrett-Mayer, E., and Wendler, D. (2006). The accuracy of surrogate decision makers a systematic review. *Archives of Internal Medicine*, **166**(5), 493–7.

Shickle, D. (1997). Public preferences for health care: Prioritisation in the United Kingdom. *Bioethics*, **11**(3–4), 277–90.

Shuster, E. (1997). Fifty years later: The significance of the Nuremberg Code. *New England Journal of Medicine*, **337**(20), 1436–40.

Siddique, R., Ricci, J. A., Stewart, W. F., *et al.* (2002). Quality of life in a U.S. national sample of adults with diabetes and motility-related upper gastrointestinal symptoms. *Digestive Diseases and Sciences*, **47**(4), 683–9.

Sieck, W. R., and Arkes, H. R. (2005). The recalcitrance of overconfidence and its contribution to decision aid neglect. *Journal of Behavioral Decision Making*, **18**(1), 29–53.

Slovic, P., Fischoff, B., Lichtenstein, S., *et al.*(1981). Perceived risk: Psychological factors and social implications (and discussion). *Proceedings of the Royal Society of London. Series A, Mathematical and Physical Sciences*, **376**(1764), 17–34.

Smith, D. M., Sherriff, R. L., Damschroder, L., *et al.* (2006). Misremembering colostomies? Former patients give lower utility ratings than do current patients. *Health Psychology*, **25**(6), 688–95.

Sonnenberg, F. A., and Beck, J. R. (1993). Markov models in medical decision making: A practical guide. *Medical Decision Making*, **13**(4), 322.

Stalmeier, P., Chapman, G. B., de Boer, A., *et al.* (2001). A fallacy of the multiplicative QALY model for low-quality weights in students and patients judging hypothetical health states. *International Journal of Technology Assessment in Health Care*, **17**(4), 488–96.

Stalmeier, P. F. M. (2002). Discrepancies between chained and classic utilities induced by anchoring with occasional adjustments. *Medical Decision Making*, **22**(1), 53–64.

Stange, K. C. (2007). Time to ban direct-to-consumer prescription drug marketing. *Annals of Family Medicine*, **5**(2), 101–4.

Stewart, T. R., Roebber, P. J., and Bosart, L. F. (1997). The importance of the task in analyzing expert judgment. *Organizational Behavior and Human Decision Processes*, **69**(3), 205–19.

Stiggelbout, A. M., Elstein, A. S., Molewijk, B., *et al.*(2006). Clinical ethical dilemmas: Convergent and divergent views of two scholarly communities. *Journal of Medical Ethics*, **32**(7), 381–8.

Straus, S. E. (2002). Individualizing treatment decisions: The likelihood of being helped or harmed. *Evaluation & the Health Professions*, **25**(2), 210–24.

Straus, S. E., Richardson, S. R., Glasziou, P., *et al.* (2005). *Evidence-based medicine: How to practice and teach EBM*, 3rd edn. Edinburgh: Churchill Livingstone.

Sutherland, H. J., Llewellyn-Thomas, H. A., Boyd, N. F., *et al.* (1982). Attitudes towards quality of survival: The concept of maximal endurable time. *Medical Decision Making*, **2**(3), 299–309.

Teigen, K., and Brun, W. (1999). The directionality of verbal probability expressions: Effects on decisions, predictions, and probabilistic reasoning. *Organizational Behavior and Human Decision Processes*, **80**(2), 155–90.

Torrance, G. W., Thomas, W. H., and Sackett, D. L. (1972). A utility maximization method for evaluation of health care programs. *Health Services Research*, **7**, 118–33.

Tversky, A., and Kahneman, D. (1974). Judgment under uncertainty: Heuristics and biases. *Science*, **185**(4157), 1124.

Tversky, A., and Kahneman, D. (1981). The framing of decisions and the psychology of choice. *Science*, **211**(4481), 453.

Tversky, A., and Kahneman, D. (1983). Extensional versus intuitive reasoning: The conjunction fallacy in probability judgment. *Psychological Review*, **90**(4), 293–315.

Tversky, A., and Kahneman, D. (1992). Advances in prospect theory: Cumulative representation of uncertainty. *Journal of Risk and Uncertainty*, **5**(4), 297–323.

Tversky, A., and Koehler, D. J. (1994). Support theory: A nonextensional representation of subjective probability. *Psychological Review*, **101**(4), 547–67.

U.S. Department of Health, Education, and Welfare. (1979). *The Belmont Report: Ethical principles and guidelines for the protection of human subjects of research.* Retrieved August 15,2007, from http://www.hhs.gov/ohrp/humansubjects/guidance/belmont.htm.

Ubel, P. A., DeKay, M. L., Baron, J., *et al.* (1996). Cost-effectiveness analysis in a setting of budget constraints: Is it equitable? *New England Journal of Medicine*, **334**(18), 1174–7.

van Ryn, M., and Burke, J. (2000). The effect of patient race and socio-economic status on physicians' perceptions of patients. *Social Science & Medicine*, **50**(6), 813–28.

Voltaire (1772). *La bégueule: conte moral* [sn].

von Neumann, J., and Morgenstern, O. (1953). *Theory of Games and Economic Behavior*. New York: John Wiley.

Von Winterfeldt, D., and Edwards, W. (1986). *Decision Analysis and Behavioral Research*. Cambridge, MA: Cambridge University Press.

Wagstaff, A. (1991). QALYs and the equity-efficiency trade-off. *Journal of Health Economics*, **10**(1), 21–41.

Wallsten, T. S. (1981). Physician and medical student bias in evaluating diagnostic information. *Medical Decision Making*, **1**(2), 145–64.

Ware, J. E., Kosinski, M., Dewey, J. E., *et al.* (2001). *How to score and interpret single-item health status measures: A manual for users of the SF-8 Health Survey*. Lincoln, RI: Quality-Metric Incorporated.

Ware, J. E., Snow, K. K., Kosinski, M., *et al.* (1993). *SF-36 Health Survey: Manual and Interpretation Guide*. Boston: The Health Institute, New England Medical Center.

Ware, J. E., Jr., and Sherbourne, C. D. (1992). The MOS 36-item short-form health survey (SF-36). I. Conceptual framework and item selection. *Medical Care*, **30**(6), 473–83.

Wear, S. (2004). Informed consent. In *Handbook of Bioethics: Taking Stock of the Field from a Philosophical Perspective*, ed. G. Khushf. Dordrecht: Kluwer Academic, pp. 251–90.

Weber, E. U., Blais, A. R., and Betz, N. E. (2002). A domain-specific risk-attitude scale: Measuring risk perceptions and risk behaviors. *Journal of Behavioral Decision Making*, **15**(4), 263–90.

Weber, E. U., Böckenholt, U. L. F., Hilton, D. J., *et al.* (2000). Confidence judgments as expressions of experienced decision conflict. *Risk, Decision and Policy*, **5**(01), 69–100.

Weinstein, M. C., Fineberg, H. V., and Elstein, A. S. (1980). *Clinical Decision Analysis*. Philadelphia, PA: Saunders.

Wenger, N. K., and Furberg, C. D. (1990). Cardiovascular disorders. In *Quality of Life Assessments in Clinical Trials*. New York: Raven Press, pp. 335–45.

Williams, A. (1997). Intergenerational equity: An exploration of the "fair innings" argument. *Health Economics*, **6**(2), 117–32.

Wilson, P. W. F., D'Agostino, R. B., Levy, D., *et al.* (1998). Prediction of coronary heart disease using risk factor categories. *Circulation*, **97**(18), 1837–47.

Wolf, F. M., Gruppen, L. D., and Billi, J. E. (1985). Differential diagnosis and the competing-hypotheses heuristic: A practical approach to judgment under uncertainty and Bayesian probability. *Journal of the American Medical Association*, **253**(19), 2858–62.

Yaniv, I. (2004). The benefit of additional opinions. *Current Directions in Psychological Science*, **13**(2), 75–7.

Yokota, F., and Thompson, K. M. (2004). Value of information literature analysis: A review of applications in health risk management. *Medical Decision Making*, **24**, 287–98.

Zaner, R. (2004). Physicians and patients in relation. In *Handbook of Bioethics: Taking Stock of the Field from a Philosophical Perspective*, ed. G. Khushf. Dordrecht: Kluwer Academic, pp. 223–50.

Zink, S., Wertlieb, S., Catalano, J., *et al.* (2005). Examining the potential exploitation of UNOS policies. *American Journal of Bioethics*, **5**(4), 6–10.

Index

Page numbers followed by t indicates tables, f indicates figures and n indicates footnotes.